CW00796420

Home Exercises For Women: Bodyweight Workouts for Women

By David Nordmark

Copyright © 2010 David Nordmark

Discover other fitness titles by David Nordmark:

Stretching Exercise Bible

Lose Weight Without Dieting

Power Isometrics

Animal Workouts

Push Up For Everyone

Stretching For Golfers

Back Stretching

Build Muscle Without Weights

Disclaimer

The exercises and advice contained within this course may be too strenuous or dangerous for some people, and the reader(s) should consult a physician before engaging in them. The author and publisher of this course are not responsible in any manner whatsoever for any injury which may occur through reading and following the instructions herein.

For More Information

If you are interested in the ideas found in this book please visit the following sites for more information.

My original website:

http://www.animal-kingdom-workouts.com/

This was the first website I ever created. It has a lot of great information but was difficult to maintain.

My natural fitness blog:

http://naturalfitness76.com/

I set up this blog as it is so much easier to update as compared to the website.

And finally, on Facebook:

https://www.facebook.com/pages/Animal-Kingdom-Workouts/610650132375018?sk=timeline

Hey, everyone's on Facebook, why not?

Table Of Contents

How I Became A Bodyweight Fitness Convert   7

Introduction To The Exercises   15

The "Holy Trilogy" - The Foundation

Of *Natural Fitness*   19

The Holy Trilogy Beginner   27

The Holy Trilogy Intermediate   35

The Holy Trilogy – Advanced   43

Additional Exercises   55

Pushup Variations   56

Squat Variations   70

Back Bending Variations   82

Additional Exercises   90

Workout Routines   142

Cardiovascular Exercises   150

About The Author   153

About The Models   154

One Last Thing   155

Also By David Nordmark   156

How I Became A Bodyweight Fitness Convert

It is my firm belief that any animal you can think of is far stronger and healthier than any human being. What's more they get this way without performing any of the exercises that man has dreamed up. A gorilla possesses super human strength, for example, yet you never see him lifting weights. A lion possesses great strength and endurance as well, yet you never see him running on a treadmill. I think there is a lesson in here for all of us. If you want to be in animal-like shape, I think it makes sense to train like they do - using nothing but your own body and bodyweight.

My own personal journey which enabled me to come to this conclusion has been a long and winding one to be sure. It was in high school that I first started to get really interested in health and fitness. I wanted to get in shape for basketball so I bought one of those Weider home gyms. Maybe you remember them. The barbells were made of plastic and you could generally find them advertised in the back of the Sears catalog. At any rate I started to work out, lifting weights and running. I thought this was the way to get in shape and I was on my way.

I'm not sure when my faith in weightlifting and running started to wane, but I can remember a few instances:

When I was still in high school using the plastic weight set, I remember once trying to do a handstand. With full confidence I kicked up into it ... and promptly collapsed in a heap in the corner. "Oh well," I thought, "I just need to get stronger." Well, I kept lifting my plastic weights and I seemed to be getting stronger. Six months later, I tried the same handstand. The result? Same as before, I collapsed in the corner. It was like my previous six months of training didn't happen at all. As I lay there in a heap looking at my ceiling I remember thinking to myself, "Hmmmm, this is weird - why aren't I stronger ...?"

Eventurally I moved on from the plastic weights and I started going to Gold's Gym. One day I was doing a leg press without too much weight at all when I felt my entire lower back move. When I say move, it felt like all of the bones there momentarily jumped an inch before they settled back down again. Basically, bones moved that really shouldn't have. Despite the fact that I was doing the exercise properly I had managed to really hurt my back. I had a hard time moving around for awhile and I still can't bend my lower back properly to this day.

From there I signed up for a Judo course in university. I really enjoyed it except for the fact that I kept getting injured. Why was I so injury prone? I used the gym regularly. Shouldn't that help? Nonetheless, it didn't. I was constantly pulling muscles in my shoulders, chest, and arms. What was going on?

After university I decided to try yoga (something I do to this day, btw) and I remember my first class vividly. In yoga you typically hold various postures for between 30 and 60 seconds. You don't use weights at all, just your own bodyweight. Well, I remember some of those simple postures were absolutely brutal. I just couldn't do it. I remember looking at some of the girls in the class, most of them looked like they hardly had any muscle in their legs at all. Nonetheless they could hold these postures with ease. Whereas myself, who regularly did exercises like squats and leg presses, couldn't do them at all.

As far as running goes, I ran pretty consistently from high school to a few years after university. Two incidents stand out in my mind. One of them was playing indoor soccer for the first time. From all the running I was doing, I figured I'd have cardio to spare. However, within minutes I was just gassed. All the long distance running I was doing didn't help me here.

The other incident is pretty obvious and pretty much ended my running days. I was still jogging but my knees were hurting more and more. I went to the doctor to get x-rays which revealed I had moderate arthritis in my right knee! All the running I had done had literally worn down the cartilage to the point that my knees were similar to that of a 70 year old man (not good when you're in your early 30's!)

It was at this time that I finally started to put things together (yeah, I know...I can be a slow learner). I started to do my own research and I started to really think for myself as to why I was doing various things fitness-wise. No longer was I going to blindly accept the received wisdom from the fitness industry. Did lifting weights make sense? I'd seriously hurt my back doing it and in any given sport I was not nearly as strong as I thought I should be. As far as running goes the soccer experience demonstrated that my cardio wasn't that great and I'd managed to severely damage my knees in the process.

This is when I really started to think about the way animals train. No animal that I know of jogs but nonetheless when needed, the endurance they possess is unbelievable. Same thing with weight training. Although they don't lift weights, the bodyweight strength animals possess is astounding.

I started doing my own research into bodyweight training in all its forms. I found that the more I trained naturally using only bodyweight workouts, the better I felt. This led me to dropping weight lifting entirely from my training routine and I've never looked back.

Based on my experience I would strenuously argue that bodyweight exercises are vastly superior to any recent "man made" exercises. This includes free weights, all workout machines, as well as all of the gimmicky exercise devices out there on the market. Why do I believe that bodyweight training is so far superior to man made forms of exercise? Let me count the ways:

- Bodyweight training works your entire body as a unit. When you perform an exercise, like the Hindu Pushup, your entire body is worked. To demonstrate this let's say your arm muscles are quite strong but your back muscles are weak. When you perform this pushup it will be your back that will get most of the work, which is exactly as it should be. Bodyweight exercises like pushups build up the strength in your body evenly. Your body works as an integrated system. When one muscle group is significantly stronger than another you are going to be that much more injury prone. This is why my body was so susceptible to injury when I was doing Judo. When you train your whole body you are building it up evenly. This is the way mother nature intended it.
- Bodyweight workouts build strength, endurance and flexibility all at the same time. The endurance factor is one that really stands out for me. Training with weights trains your muscles to give bursts of strength but only for

10

a short time. When you train naturally you'll build real bodyweight strength which equals power plus endurance. This is really something you'll have to experience for yourself. The person who can do 10 squats with weight will not be able to do 100 (much less 500) hindu squats in a row. The person who does hindu squats will be able to do the 10 weighted squats with ease.

- Bodyweight workout routines will melt fat off your body like nobody's business. Training with your whole body allows you to use the maximum number of muscles at any one time. It's simple. The more muscles you work, the more calories you'll burn. This is the exact opposite of weight training which only works small groups of muscles.
- You are much less likely to get injured. Go on the internet right now and google "running injuries" or "weight lifting injuries". When you do so you will find entire web pages dedicated to these topics. The problem is that man did not evolve lifting weights. He evolved just like our animal brothers did, working with his own body and bodyweight. When he deviates from this he gets into trouble.
- Bodyweight fitness programs work your entire body from the inside out. Old time fitness pioneers always emphasized the importance of training your internal organs. If these were not healthy you were not healthy, no matter what your outer appearance would indicate. All of the bodyweight exercises you are about to learn involve deep breathing and many of them provide gentle massages for your internal

organs. The health benefits from these are enormous.

- Bodyweight exercises not only build your muscles but also your joints and ligaments, as well. Weight lifting, particularly with heavy weights, puts strain on your joints and ligaments which wear them down. When you train naturally with your own bodyweight, your joints and ligaments get stronger with you.

- Bodyweight training accentuates a man's masculinity and a women's femininity. I know this is an unusual one at first glance so let me explain. Men and women are different and I think it's fair to say that they want different results from any kind of exercise program they engage in. Men typically want to get larger and stronger whereas women, although they want to get stronger, do not want to look like a man with giant muscles. When you train naturally, you are working with Mother Nature, as well as, the ying and yang of your inner being. Men will get bigger and stronger. Women however, although they'll be performing the exact same exercises, will get that 'fit and sexy', strong yet feminine look. Training naturally allows a man to be a man and a woman to be a woman, which is how it should be.

Through trial and error and by trying almost every bodyweight exercise I could, I eventually came to the following conclusion: if you want to possess animal-like strength and endurance you need to do three exercises. You need to perform an exercise to work your lower body, an exercise to work your upper body, and an exercise to work your spine and back. I call these three exercises the holy trilogy of bodyweight training and I'll get to more detail about them in a moment. Just know for now that if you do these three exercises - at a minimum - you'll be in great shape. It is these three exercises that form the foundation for this book.

Introduction to the Exercises

Who can perform these exercises?

Anyone in good health who has no pre-existing medical conditions and has their doctor's approval to begin an exercise program. Men and women of all ages (40's, 50's, 60's) will benefit from this program, as well as children.

How long should I exercise?

As a general rule of thumb 15 minutes a day is all you need. In the beginning you are most likely going to have trouble performing even 5 hindu pushups or 10 hindu squats (I know I did). You will most likely find that 15 minutes is plenty.

How often should I exercise?

I would recommend that you aim to exercise everyday. You are far better off exercising for 15 minutes a day everyday than performing 1 hour workouts 3 times a week. Do you shower everyday? Do you brush your teeth? You should approach exercise the same way for the maximum benefits. However, I do realize that the simple demands of life sometimes make this impossible. You'll still get great results if you exercise four or five times a week.

How many repetitions/sets should I do?

For all of the exercises I give general guidelines as to how many repetitions you should do. However, keep in mind these are only guidelines. You have a brain, don't be afraid to use it! If you are getting the results you want by performing 100 hindu squats and 50 hindu pushups in one go then stick with it. If you're not an athlete this is really all you need to do to look fantastic and be fit. On the other hand, if you are an athlete of some kind or you just want to get in super shape then the sky's really the limit as to the number of repetitions you can do. It's possible to perform 500 hindu squats in under 15 minutes. You can perform 250 hindu pushups if you want to. There are people out there who do this and more. It's really up to you. You know your body and, more importantly, you know what you want. Do what works for you.

As far as sets go I recommend performing one set for all of these exercises. Performing sets (doing the same exercise for a number of reps, resting, then doing it again) is really a holdover from the bodybuilder mentality. With bodyweight training you want to build strength and endurance. Animals don't train in sets and neither should you. Do the maximum number of reps you can for any given exercise then move on to the next one. This has the added benefit of being more interesting, as well.

How should I train?

When exercising focus on your breathing and what you are doing. Do not train with the music blaring in the background or with the television on. Concentrate on the movements. You'll make much faster progress this way.

Do I need to watch what I eat?

If you want to maximize your results – yes. For starters I suggest you track down my ebook, "Lose Weight WITHOUT Dieting". This book contains some straightforward advice on how to change your eating habits in order to lose weight for the long term. Diets don't work but using your mind to change your long term eating habits does. If you want to get in the best shape of your life you need to focus on exercise and what you eat. You could exercise everyday for hours but if your eating habits are poor, you will not get the results you want.

If you are looking to really take it to another level another program you might want to check out is Tom Venuto's "Burn The Fat / Feed The Muscle" program. Tom's a natural bodybuilder and I'm not big on bodybuilding. However, the one thing bodybuilders know how to do is to eat properly to maximize fat loss and muscle growth. If you want to look like a fitness model or a close approximation, it's worth your time to check out his program. You can find it here:

http://tinyurl.com/burnfatprogram

What clothing and equipment do I need?

As far as clothes are concerned whatever you are most comfortable wearing. Shorts and an old T shirt work fine. In the pictures the models are wearing shoes but you don't even need those. Training in your bare feet helps to strengthen them and this is how I often train. Beyond that, you just need a room with a little bit of free space and perhaps a towel or a small exercise mat. From there you're good to go.

How do I start?

Great question! For me it begins with what I consider to be the "Holy Trilogy" of bodyweight exercises. This means that each workout should contain some form of an...a) pushup b) squat and c) back bending. This "Holy Trilogy" forms the foundation for the Home Exercises program. Why is this? Read on to learn why!

The "Holy Trilogy" - The Foundation Of Natural Fitness

Pushups, squats and back bending make up the foundation of the Home Exercises bodyweight fitness program. The reason for this is that by doing all three, you are simultaneously stretching and strengthening your entire body all at once. In fact, if you just performed these three exercises daily in moderation (you could get a great workout done in under 15 minutes) you'd be in better shape than 95% of the population. Let's look at each exercise in a little more detail to learn why they are so important.

Pushups

The pushup is a bodyweight exercise that really needs no introduction. Who, at some point in time, hasn't done a pushup? This classic exercise works the entire body (including your legs) but is particularly focused on the upper body. Nothing works your chest, back and arms like the pushup. Below are some other benefits of pushups you may not be aware off.

- They utilize the three types of muscle building at the same time. These are concentric (muscle is stimulated to contract), eccentric (muscle elongates due to contraction of another muscle) and isometric (the muscle attempts to contract but does not actually change in length).
- They can help improve your reaction time by training your proprioceptive muscle fibers. These fibers are the microscopic nerves that keep your body balanced. When you perform a pushup these nerves have to constantly fire to keep yourself from tipping over. This trains them to respond quickly to stimulation, which will aide your balance and speed.
- Performing pushups in high reps encourages blood flow. Often when you exert yourself, either by playing a sport or just general work, your muscles will start to feel sore due to the buildup of lactic acid in them. The blood flow that pushups encourage actually help minimize this effect by flushing out the affected areas.
- They'll simply make you stronger with greater muscular endurance. But you knew that, right?

Squats

Bodyweight squats are like pushups for your lower body. All of the benefits I mentioned for pushups above can be applied to squats, as well. In addition, performing bodyweight squats also has the following benefits:

- Your legs contain the largest muscles in your body. When you work them with high rep squats, you will burn fat like crazy. Who doesn't want this?
- Squats will help keep you young. When elite athletes lose their edge what do they lose first? Their legs. It doesn't matter whether it's a boxer, basketball player or runner. Now you may not be any of these - but it doesn't matter. Being able to simply walk with pep and vigor is a sign of youth. Bodyweight squats will help you maintain this.
- Helps to keep your heart healthy. I was once at a yoga seminar where the speaker made the point that healthy legs can act like a second heart for your lower body. When people get older and start having trouble with their circulation where do the problems often start? In their legs. Strong healthy legs make it easier for your heart to pump blood. Doesn't this sound beneficial?
- Squats, particularly when done in high reps, will help you build endurance and lung power.

Back Bending

As important as pushups and squats are, neither of them are as critical to your health as performing some kind of exercise which works your spine. Think about it. You can hurt your leg and still hobble around if you need to. You can hurt an arm and still function. When you hurt your back, however, you instantaneously become an old man or women. A sore back can make a simple task, like getting up from a chair, nearly impossible. "A healthy spine leads to a healthy life" is a common saying in yoga. But how exactly do we work our spines? The answer: by performing exercises which involve back bending.

To understand why this is so you need to look at the human spine from an evolutionary perspective. Evolution is a clunky process. When a creature is forced to adapt to a changing environment it does not start with a clean slate. It must adapt whatever systems it already has as best it can. In our case, our human spines evolved when we were still walking on all fours. This means our spines were ideally adapted to carry an even load along its entire length.

When human beings started to walk on two legs this all changed. Rather than having the weight of the body distributed evenly, the spine was now vertical. In a way the modern human spine resembles a flag pole with a large weight (the head) on the very top. This puts tremendous strain on the back (paricularly the lower back) and is one of the main reasons so many of us experience back pain.

When this basic structural flaw is combined with a modern lifestyle which often involves activities such as slouching forward, staring at computers or driving long distances, you have problems. These activities all conspire to put a tremendous strain on an already compromised system, the back.

When you perform a back bend you're are doing two things. The first thing you are doing is relieving the tension that naturally builds up in your back throughout the day (especially if you're sitting). The back is meant to move in all directions but most of us only bend forwards. Back bending helps correct this. The second thing you are doing is strengthening the muscles along the back and spine. Stronger back muscles are obviously important when it comes to supporting the spine and thereby, avoiding pain.

In Conclusion

When you combine pushups, squats and back bending together you will be getting a full body workout that will simultaneously increase your strength, flexibility and endurance. What follows now are three different versions (basic, intermediate and advanced) of "The Holy Trilogy". I suggest you start at a level that you feel comfortable with. As you get better you can either simply increase the number of reps you are doing for a particular exercise or replace it with a more difficult version. Once you have reached the advanced level, you can add on more exercises as you see fit. However, I urge you to never completely forget about the Holy Trilogy. Every exercise session you do should incorporate some form of a pushup, squat and back bend.

One Final Note - Are Bodyweight Squats Safe?

One of the biggest controversies I've come across in the bodyweight community is the question of whether performing squats are safe for the knees. The argument that is made is that some squats, like Hindu Squats, are dangerous because your knees go over your toes and this "shears the knees". Is this true?

I've looked into this and have yet to find one scientific study that actually backs up this claim. If I'm wrong, please write me and let me know where to find the study. I'd love to take a look at it.

In my opinion, squatting is a natural human movement and should be trained as such. Think about it. If you were not supposed to be able to squat down with your back relatively straight while coming up on your toes with your knees extending past your toes, you wouldn't be able to do it.

For thousands of years human beings existed without furniture and would often squat down and perform a myriad of activities from this position. This is still true in large parts of the world today. In Asia, huge numbers of people sit like this (knees extended over toes) for long periods of time. If this position destroyed your knees it seems to me that knee problems would be a common issue in Asia. The reality is that Asians, on average, have far healthier knees and backs than North Americans.

Another example I'll point out is the Great Gama. The Great Gama was a world champion wrestler, when professional wrestling was a real sport, at the turn of the last century. He would perform between 500 and 1000 Hindu Squats, or Dands, a day. Did he have knee problems? Far from it. He was one of the strongest and best conditioned athletes of his day and he never suffered from knee problems.

When people start performing deep knee squats, they may at first experience some discomfort in the knees, as your body will need time to strengthen the tendons and ligament in the knees, not to mention the muscles. This discomfort typically goes away after about four weeks.

Now, having said all of the above, I would add one caveat. You know your body better than anyone else. If you try Hindu Squats or some variant and experience knee pain that doesn't go away...stop doing it. Use your common sense. In these situations, I would recommend bringing your thighs down to a point where they are parallel to the floor and no deeper. By doing so you will still be getting the benefits and you'll be strengthening your knees at the same time. You can try performing the squat more deeply in the future or simply stick with the parallel thigh version. Always remember that you do have a brain. Don't be afraid to use it!

Now with that out of the way let's move on to the exercises!

The Holy Trilogy Beginner

If you are a complete beginner to bodyweight exercises I suggest you start here. The beginner holy trilogy is made up of combo pushups, boot strappers and ying yang bends. Try to do these exercises everyday if possible. I suggest doing them first thing in the morning before you go to work. They can be done in under 15 minutes and will get you in a great mood for the day ahead. When you can perform 20 combo pushups, 50 boot strappers and 10 standing back bends it's probably time to move onto the intermediate level.

Combo Pushups

Many people find that even performing one classic pushup to be beyond their abilities. If this is the case, then the Combo Pushup is for you. By lowering yourself down in a full pushup, you will be strengthening your entire body and training yourself to perform the full pushup. Pressing back up on your knees is what separates this exercise from the Classic. Once you can do 20 it is a good idea to move onto the Classic Pushup.

1. Lie down on the floor and get into the classic pushup position.
2. Cross both of your ankles in the air, bending at the knees.
3. Exhale through your nose as you press up.
4. Once you are at the top, uncross your ankles and straighten your legs. You should now be in the full pushup position. Inhale through your nose and lower yourself to the floor.
5. Once you are on the floor cross your ankles again and press up as a knee pushup.

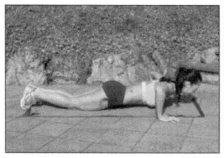 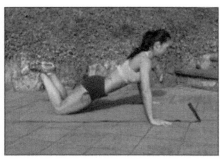

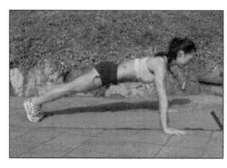 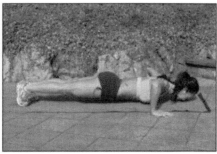

Bootstrappers

This bodyweight squat variation is ideal for beginners - as the hands provide stability while taking some of the body's weight, as well. Make sure you keep your stomach tight when you perform this exercise to protect your lower back. If you feel any strain in your lower back, it is acceptable to keep your knees slightly bent in the "Up" position.

1. Begin by squatting down with your knees together and your heels off the floor.
2. Lean forward and put your hands on the ground just in front of your shoulders. Make sure your toes are pointed forward. 60% of your weight should be on your legs and 40% on your hands.
3. Straighten your legs until your heels touch the ground.
4. Bend your legs and return to the starting position in #1.

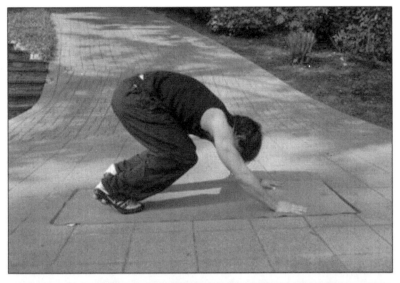

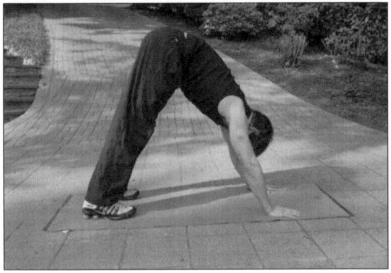

31

Ying/Yang Bends

1. Begin standing with your feet shoulder width apart and your knees slightly bent. Place your hands on the back of your hips / lower back for support.
2. Look up at the ceiling and breathe in through your nose as you bend your back backwards. Go as far as you can while maintaining your balance. Imagine that you are trying to look at the wall behind you.
3. Bend forward at the waist while exhaling your breath through your nose. Touch your hands to the floor. If you have trouble reaching the floor, it is OK to bend your knees more.
4. Repeat this motion 10 times.

Additional Notes

Remember to go slowly and deliberately. Don't rush anything.

Keep your knees slightly bent and your stomach tight at all times. This takes pressure off the lower back.

This exercise is great for the lower back, spine and waist.

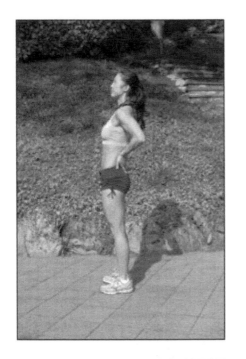
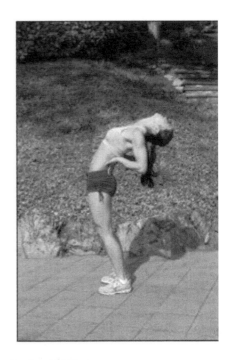
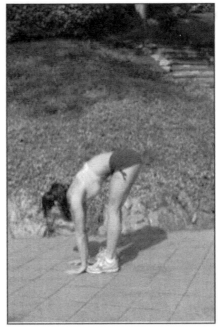

The Holy Trilogy Intermediate

Once you're comfortable performing the beginner Holy Trilogy, it's time to move onto the intermediate exercises. These include the classic pushup, personal power squats and the cobra. Once you can perform 20 classic pushups and 50 squats you can start thinking about moving on to the advanced level.

Classic Floor Pushups

1. Lie down with your stomach on the floor and your legs straight behind you.
2. Put your arms in the 90/90 pushup position.
3. Take a deep breath through your nose and then start to exhale as you press yourself up off the floor.
4. Inhale through your nose as you lower yourself back onto the floor.

Additional Notes

Remember to keep your back straight with your abdominals and glutes contracted at all times.

The 90/90 pushup position refers to the starting position for a pushup. To get into it lie down on the floor with your arms straight out from your sides. Your arms and body should be at a 90 degree angle to each other. Now bend your arms at the elbows at 90 degrees. Rotate your arms at the shoulders until the palms of your hands are underneath your elbows. You are now ready to perform a pushup.

If your wrists bother you at all, feel free to adjust your hand position to eliminate this feeling.

Another option is to put your hands into a "fist" position with your knuckles on the ground. This will completely eliminate the bend in your wrist. You may want to place a towel under your knuckles for comfort, however.

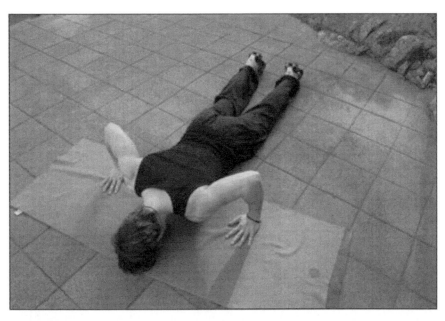

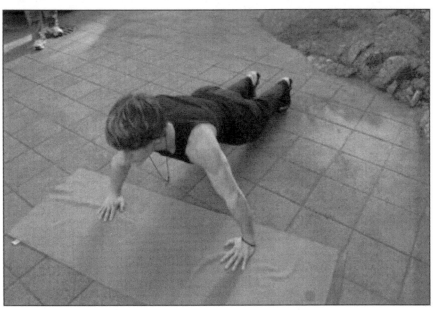

Personal Power Squats

If your knees bother you, you may want to try these before you attempt the hindu squats. They really work the quadriceps muscles, which are located at the front of your thighs. Do these slowly, holding onto a chair or desk for support, if needed.

1. Stand straight with one of your hands resting on a chair.
2. Keeping your back as straight as possible, slowly start to bend your knees, lowering your butt to the ground. Try and keep your back as straight and perpendicular to the ground as possible.
3. Try and lower yourself to the point that your thighs are almost parallel to the floor. If you have poor knees simply go as far as you are comfortable. Reach forward with your other hand to maintain balance, if needed.
4. Pause for a moment then stand up straight again. This constitutes one rep.

Again, try and keep your back as straight as you can and perpendicular to the ground. One thought that might help you here is to imagine the way you would arch your back if someone were to drop an ice cube down it. This is how straight you will want your back at all times. This motion should be done slowly and deliberately. Aim for doing between 25 and 50 reps.

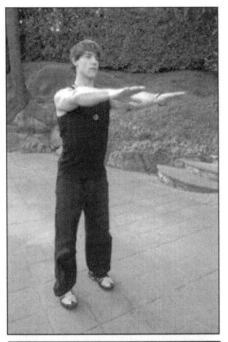 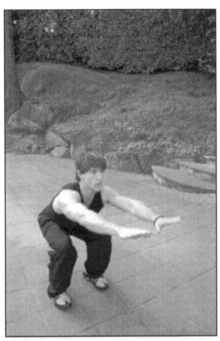

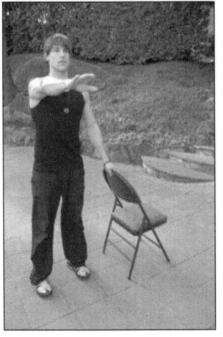 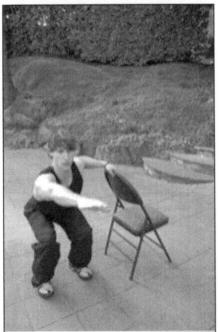

Cobra Posture

Cobra's are known to have the strongest spines in the world. By performing this posture, so will you!

1. Begin by lying on the ground with your heals together. Your eyes should be looking forward, not at the ground.
2. Place your palms on the ground close to your shoulders.
3. Squeeze your butt tightly and use your back muscles to lift your chest off the ground. If needed, you can use your arms to assist you. However, remember that this is not a pushup. Overtime you will want to transfer the workload away from your arms so that your back and butt are getting most of the workout. Tilt your head backward and look upward. This will raise your stomach off the ground. Your hips should stay on the ground throughout the entire movement.

This exercise will stretch your stomach and relieve tension from your back. Take it easy when first performing this stretch as most people are not used to back bending. Try to hold the posture for 10 seconds, working your way up to 30.

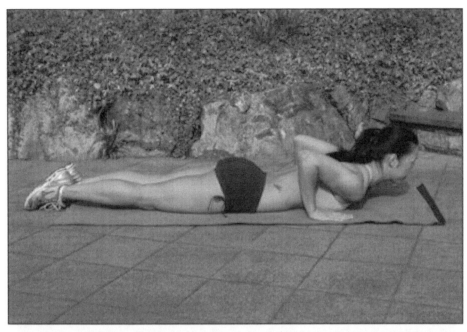

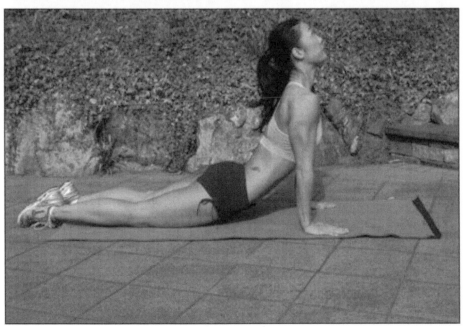

The Holy Trilogy – Advanced

The hindu squat, pushup and back bridge are the exercises I started with many years ago. The sky is really the limit with these. The Great Gama reportedly used to do 500 hindu squats and 250 hindu pushups a day. There's no need for you to do this. If you perform 100 hindu squats, 50 hindu pushups and hold the bridge for a minute, you'll be in fantastic shape. Once you've performed these exercises for about a month, you can start adding some of the supplementary exercises as you wish, as well as, trying some of the other pushups and squat variations.

Hindu Squats

Hindu squats are one of the most basic exercises that I try to perform every morning as they really warm up my body and get my blood pumping. You will find that hindu squats build trememdous strength and endurance in your legs while the motion of the exercise also works your back, chest, and arms. What's more, hindu squats really build your lung power. When they are performed vigorously, 5 minutes of hindu squats will have you huffing and puffing like you've just run a couple of miles. If you want to really build up your cardiovascular endurance, hindu squats beat running hands down.

The first time I tried this exercise (I was also running and weightlifting at the time) I could barely do 10. If you're like how I was don't get discouraged. Just figure out what you can do on Day 1 then work on doing just one more the next day. You can really work up to doing as many as you want. For myself as of this writing, I do 200 a day. However, some people do 500 in under 15 minutes while others do many more. You really have to decide what is right for you.

Most women I know want strong, sexy, toned legs. If this is what you want as well, then the hindu squat is the exercise you want to do. Building your leg muscles naturally will give them the shape and tone that nature intended. If you went to a gym you'd have to workout on I don't know how many machines to achieve a similar appearance and your legs still wouldn't possess the *functional* strength you get from this one bodyweight exercise.

How to Perform a Hindu Squat

1. Start with your feet shoulder-width apart and arms extended out from your chest parallel to the floor.
2. Breathe deeply, filling your lungs as you clench your fists and pull them toward your chest.
3. Keeping your back as straight as possible, lower your body by bending your knees. As you lower your body, you should extend your arms downward as well, behind your back if possible. Start to exhale the air from your lungs.
4. Toward the bottom of the movement you should come up on your toes, keeping as straight a spine as possible.
5. Straighten your legs by pushing off your toes and swinging your arms forward. As you rise, press your heels to the floor and raise your arms to chest level, parallel to the floor.

Additional Notes

You should always inhale when you pull your arms in and exhale as you lower your body.

Performed correctly, your arms should look like you're rowing a boat.

When you are lowering your body, you should try and place your hands behind your back. However, if you are tall, you may have to keep you hands at your side for balance.

Work toward keeping your back as straight as possible at all times. When you are in the standing position, arch your lower back while bringing your chest up and out and your shoulder blades back and down. It might help you to imagine how you reacted when someone put some snow down your back when you were a kid. You want to try and arch your back in the same way.

It is possible to perform a leg workout of 500 Hindu Squats in 15 minutes everyday. However, you will get great results from doing 100 daily. At first you will probably find it hard to do 25. Work at it to determine what level is right for you and your goals.

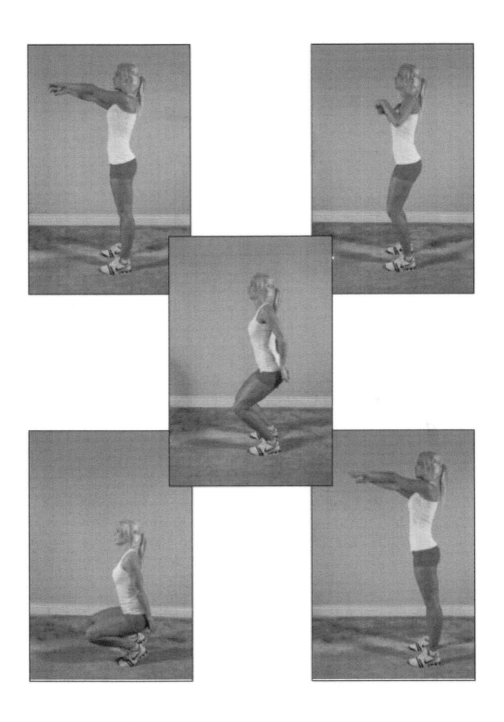

Hindu Pushups

The hindu pushup, or dand, is a bodyweight strength exercise that originated in India. Indian wrestlers, such as the Great Gama, were known to perform hundreds of them everyday which gave them great strength and stamina. Like all great bodyweight exercises, hindu pushups work your entire body including your arms, back, chest, and legs. It also massages your internal organs while increasing the flexibility of your spine, hips, and shoulders. Remember to breathe in through your nose and out through your mouth as you perform this exercise. Breathe deeply and with a powerful intent in order to really build your lung power.

How to Perform a Hindu Pushup (Dand)

1. To get into the ready position to perform a Hindu Pushup, start in the "up" position of a regular pushup, with your feet spread wider than shoulder width.
2. Walk your hands backward so that your butt is in the air, your arms and legs are straight, and you are looking back through your legs. From the side, your body should resemble an inverted "V".
3. Start bending your elbows so that your body comes forward. Your hips will come down toward the floor.
4. Before your head hits the floor start to arch your spine so that you are looking toward the ceiling. Straighten your arms and exhale while you look at the ceiling.

5. Keep your arms straight and push your butt back to position 2 while inhaling.

Additional Notes

The Great Gama would (according to legend) perform up to 250 of these a day, which shows you what is possible. Do you need to do that many? Of course not. If you work your way up to 50 a day you'll be in great shape. Don't be surprised if it takes you awhile to work up to that goal, however. The first time I tried this exercise I think I did 5. Again, take it slowly and just work on doing one more each day.

When performing this exercise make sure that you breathe deeply and that you use your mind. Don't have loud music blaring in the background. Focus on what you are doing. Imagine that you are a wave of water crashing against the shore. Your motion should be fluid, like the waves rolling on the open ocean.

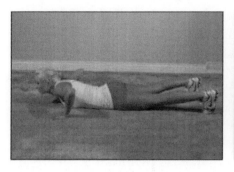 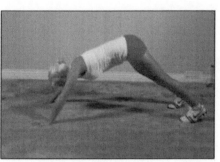

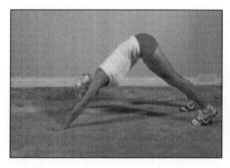 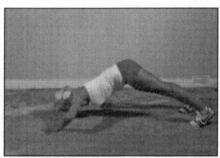

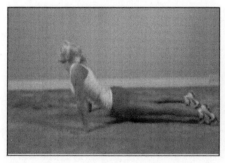 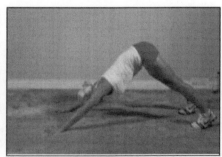

Back Bridge

The secret to remaining strong and vigorous throughout your life is a strong and healthy spine. More than any other body part, it is your back that is the key to your health. You can pull a muscle in your leg or arm and still function. If you hurt your back, however, you immediately become the equivalent of a 90 year old man or woman in poor health.

All animals in nature have extraordinarily healthy and flexible spines and can bend them in all directions. Our spines should be the same way although most of us are far from this ideal. The reason for this is that most of us in the modern world spend a great deal of time bending over computers, sitting at desks, or driving. We rarely, if ever, bend our backs backward. This is to our great detriment and one of the major reasons why so many people have back problems.

I've tried many different back exercises which involve back bending, some of which are in this book. However the best back exercise that I've found is the back bridge. Not only does it strengthen and stretch your neck and spine, it will work your entire body as well.

The first time I tried a back bridge it was a little bit scary. I was not used to bending my back backward and my neck was very weak. I remember the first time I arched my back backwards. I could feel my spine stretch and it made noises that sounded like tiny twigs snapping. Still, I persisted and I can honestly say that my back is far healthier as a result. As of this writing, I fully intend to perform some kind of back bridge everyday until the day I die. This is how much I believe in this exercise.

As with any bodyweight exercise in this book, the key is to take it slowly and do what you can do. If you can only arch backward for a split second, that's great. Just come back the next day and try and do a little bit more. I suspect you're going to be surprised at how fast your back responds to this exercise.

Preparing your Body for the Back Bridge

When you first start performing this exercise you will probably want to begin by rocking your body back and forth. Here's what to do:

1. Lie down on a soft mat or carpet with your back facing down.
2. Bend your legs so that your feet are close to your butt. Place your hands face down by your shoulders. Pushup with your legs so that you arch your back and you drive your body backward.
3. Your weight should now be supported by your feet, hands, and the top of your head. Rock backwards, rolling on your head. Your goal is to touch your nose to the mat.
4. When you can rock back and forth 20 times, touching your nose to the mat as you do so, you are ready to move on to the hand supported back bridge.

Hand Supported Back Bridge

This exercise is exactly the same as above. However, when you are able to touch your nose to the mat, you will want to hold this position for time.

1. Lie down on a soft mat with your back facing down.
2. Bend your legs so that your feet are close to your butt. Place your hands face down by your shoulders.

3. Pushup with your legs so that you arch your back, driving your body backward. Your weight should now be supported by your feet, hands, and the top of your head.
4. Drive backwards with your feet so that your nose is touching the mat. Hold it there.
5. Breathe slowly and naturally through your nose. Concentrate on your breathing and try to remain as still as possible. That will make this exercise much easier.
6. Hold this position for as long as possible. Aim for 3 minutes, which is the rough equivalent of 20 to 25 deep breaths.

Arms Folded Back Bridge

When you're comfortable performing the hand supported back bridge then you are ready to try it without hand support. The steps are the same as above except that now when you touch your nose to the mat, you'll want to fold your arms in front of your chest. Again, shoot for three minutes, although you can really hold it for as long as you want.

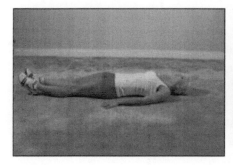 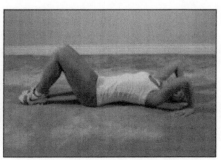

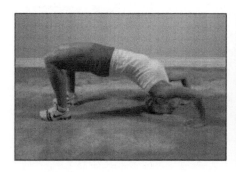 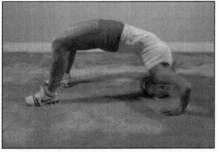

Additional Exercises

Once you feel you've mastered the holy trilogy of pushups, squats and back bending you can begin adding new exercises to your routine as you see fit. What follows are sections on pushups, squats and back bending variations as well as additional exercises that you will find interesting and challenging. Moving forward I would make the following recommendations for you:

1. Always make sure you are doing some form of a pushup, squat and backbend in every workout session. In order to keep things interesting it's fine to try the wall squat instead of the hindu squat, for example. Just make sure you are always doing some form of the holy trilogy at all times.
2. The supplementary exercises are just that, supplementary. Once you have completed at least one exercise for each of the holy trilogy you can add some of these exercises on as you see fit.

As always, take it easy. Some of the exercises that follow are somewhat easy whereas others are extremely difficult. Go at your own pace and build slowly. Remember, it's the tortoise that wins the race, not the hare. Have fun and good luck!

Pushup Variations

Walk Out Push Up

This exercise is perfect for indoor training. By itself the pushup gives you a full body workout, but you also get a "mini bear crawl" when you walk out.

1. Stand with your feet together and your arms at your sides.
2. Bend your knees into a squat and place your hands in front of you.
3. Walk forward on your hands until you are in the pushup position.
4. Perform a pushup.
5. Walk backward with you hands and return to the crouch position.
6. Stand and repeat. Continue until fatigued.

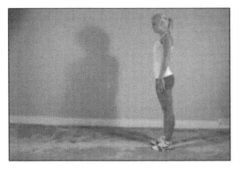
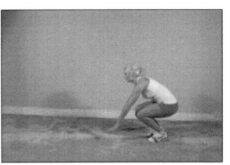

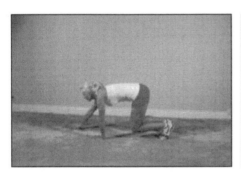
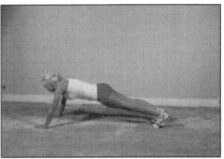

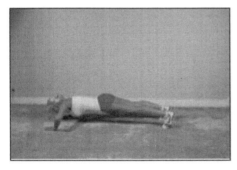
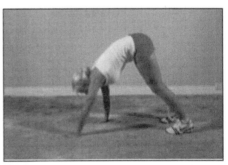

Pike Push Up

The pike push up is a great intermediate step if you want to build up the strength to perform a full hand stand push up. It really works your shoulders and arms and really gives you a sense of what it's like to work with your own bodyweight.

1. Assume the standard push up position with your feet together.
2. Walk your hands backward toward your feet so that your body resembles an inverted "V".
3. Bend your arms so that you lower your body to the floor.
4. Push back up to the starting position. Hold your body and head steady at all times.

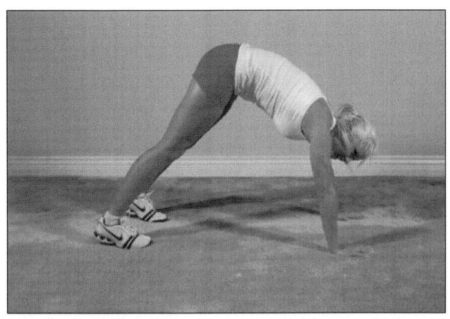

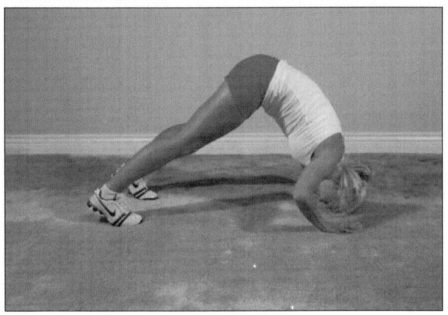

Elevated Pike Push Up

This is a more advanced and difficult version of the pike pushup. It builds real bodyweight strength in the arms and shoulders and is a great intermediate step to performing a handstand pushup.

1. Place your toes on a stable, elevated object like a chair. Assume a pushup-like position with your hands on the floor.
2. Walk your hands backward so that your legs and upper body are at right angles. Your body should now be perpendicular to the floor.
3. Lower your body toward the floor and then push back up again. Try to keep your body and head steady as you do this. Inhale as you lower you body, exhale when you pushup.

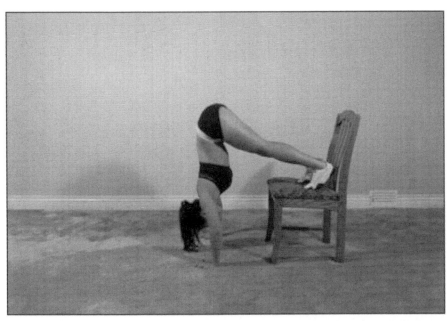

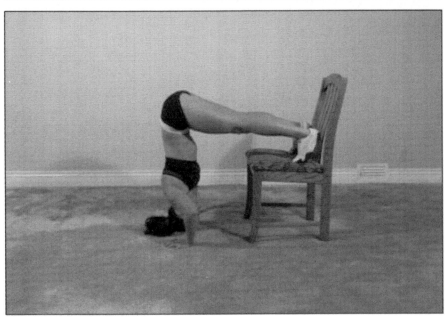

Atlas Pushups

Atlas pushups are a form of pushup popularized by the legendary Charles Atlas. In order to perform them, you will need two sturdy chairs. This exercise really works the chest, arms, and back.

1. Place two chairs side by side about 18 inches apart.
2. Place each of your hands on the seat of the chairs with your arms straight. The rest of your body should be straight as well as extended toward the floor. This is the starting position.
3. Bend your elbows and lower yourself between the chairs as far as you can go.
4. Push yourself back up to the starting position. Breathe in as you lower yourself, breathe out as you push yourself back up.
5. Try for 25 reps or until you feel slightly fatigued.

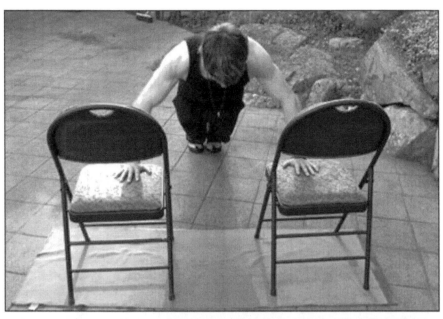

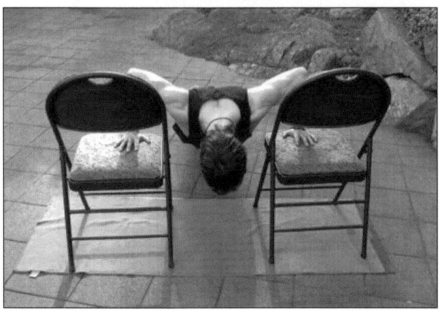

63

Reverse Pushup

The reverse pushup is a truly great bodyweight exercise. Not only does it strengthen your back, shoulders and arms, but it also promotes flexibility and suppleness in those areas, as well.

1. Lie down with your back on the floor. Bend your knees so that your feet are close to your butt and flat on the floor. Place your hands next to the top of your shoulders with your palms on the ground.
2. Push your body off the floor using your legs and arms. Attempt to straighten your arms while simultaneously arching your back. The top of your head should be facing the floor.
3. Using your legs, drive your body backwards. Try and get your chest even with your arms.
4. Slowly lower yourself to the floor. You want your upper back to touch the floor first, not your head.

Do as many repetitions of this exercise as possible. When you first try it you may not even be able to get off the ground. Do not worry about this. If this is the case just push as hard as you can. Before you know it you will be able to get your body of the ground. Remember to exhale at the top of the movement, inhale at the bottom.

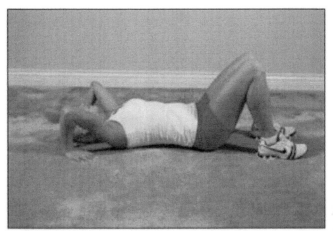

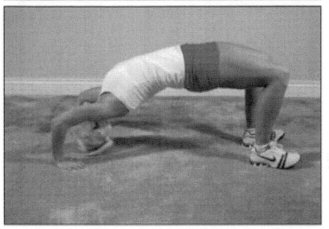

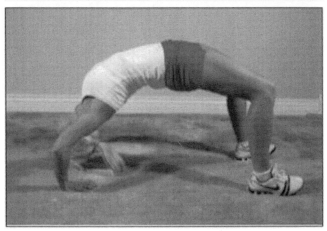

Finger Tip Pushup

The finger tip pushup gives you all of the benefits of a regular pushup while really building strength in your fingers and forearms. If you want to increase your grip strength, this is the bodyweight strength exercise to do.

1. Lie down flat on the floor with your hands palm down by your shoulders. Balance on your fingertips instead of your palms.
2. Take a deep breath. As you exhale, pushup with your arms and your fingertips.
3. Inhale as your lower yourself, lightly touching your chest to the floor. Repeat as many times as you are able.

As your fingers get stronger you will want to come up higher and higher on your fingers. When you get really strong you can start removing fingers (By removing fingers, I don't mean to cut them off! Rather, I mean you can balance on your thumb and three fingers, rather than four fingers.) to make the exercise even harder. On the other hand, if your fingers are too weak to perform even one fingertip pushup you may want to start by performing the pushup vertically against a wall instead. The further you are from the wall, the harder the exercise will be. Before long you will be able to perform the pushup on the floor.

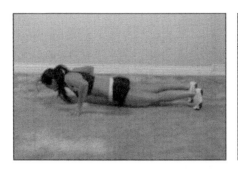
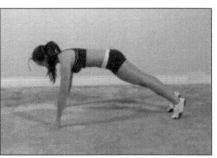
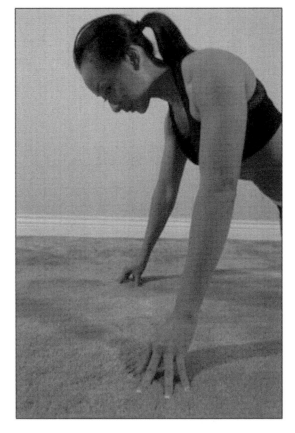

Handstand Pushups

The handstand pushup is an extremely advanced exercise that builds strength in your shoulders, back, and arms like nothing else. If you have a hard time performing a pull up, try working on your handstand pushups first. When you can do 15 full handstand pushups in a row, try performing a pull up again. I think you'll be surprised how much easier it is.

1. Place your hands on the floor about 18 inches from the wall.
2. Place your right knee under your chest.
3. Pushup up with your left leg while you simultaneously kick up with your right. Try to touch the wall with your feet as softly as you can. You don't want to put a hole in your wall.
4. You should be in a reverse handstand position with your feet resting gently against the wall.
5. Bend your elbows and lower your body so that your nose approaches the ground. Ideally, you want to be looking at the floor the whole way down until you touch your forehead to the floor.
6. Go as far as you can, then reverse direction and push back up again.

When you first try this exercise you will most likely not be able to perform one repetition. If you can't push yourself back up just keep pushing until you've had enough - which will turn the movement into an isometric exercise. When you lower yourself, you don't need to go all the way at first. If you can only lower yourself 1/4 or a 1/2 then do that. Just keep working at it.

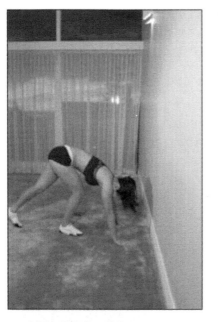 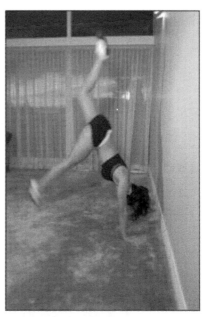

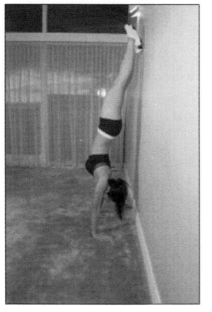 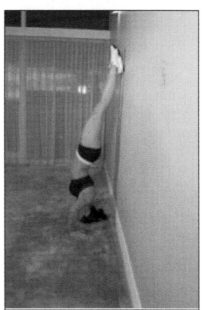

Squat Variations

Sumo Squat

1. Begin with your heels slightly wider than shoulder width apart and your toes turned out to either side almost like a clown.
2. Keeping your back straight, lower your back to the ground. Breathe in through your nose as you do so. You should feel a gentle stretch in your hips, groin and lower back.
3. Breathe in through your nose as you raise your body back to the starting position.
4. Do not rush the movement. Perform this squat 10 to 20 times.

Additional Points

Turn your toes outward as far as you can while still maintaining your balance. If your legs are really stiff simply turn them out as far as you can.

When you lower your body always look straight ahead. This will help keep your back straight.

This exercise will also promote flexibility in your inner thighs and groin.

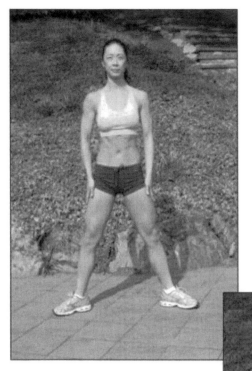

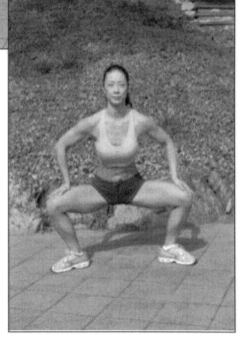

Wall Chair

This exercise is fantastic for building strength and endurance, as well. Skiers, speed skaters and hockey players often use this form of bodyweight training to build their leg strength. When performing this exercise, make sure you always concentrate on your breathing. Breathe calmly and slowly through your nose, keeping your focus on a fixed point in front of you.

1. Place your back against a wall.
2. Lower yourself so that you are sitting in an imaginary chair. Your feet should be shoulder width apart.
3. Fold your arms across your chest and relax while you breathe deeply.

Try and hold this posture for a minute. As you progress you should be able to hold this posture for longer periods of time.

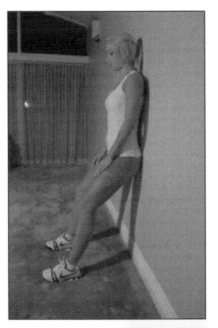
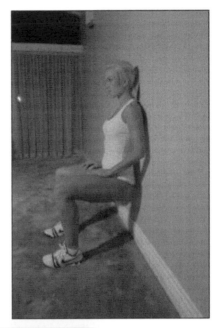
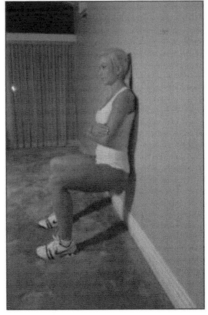

One Legged Bootstrappers

This variation on the bootstrap really works the single leg. Remember to reverse this exercise so that you work both legs.

1. Begin in the "Up" position of the regular bootstrap except this time, place your right foot on your left Achilles tendon. Your left foot should be flat on the ground.
2. Bend your left knee as far as you can into a squat. Your left heel should come off the ground.
3. Press up on your left foot and repeat.

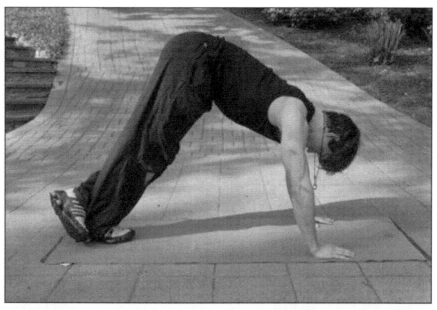

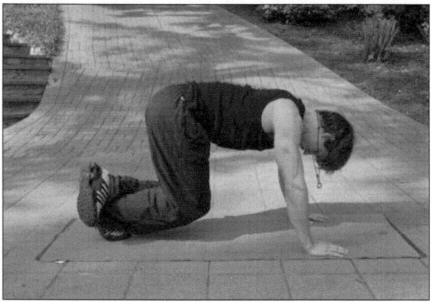

One Leg Back Squats

Once you have built up a lot of strength in your lower body you might want to give one legged squats a try. Aside from building leg strength they really work on your balance too.

1. Begin standing with your arms straight in front of you.
2. Bend one knee at 90 degrees while keeping the other one straight.
3. Begin bending the straight leg, slowly lowering your butt to the floor while keeping your back straight..
4. Lower yourself as far as you are comfortable. The maximum you want to go is to the point where your rear foot touches the ground. Return to the starting position to complete one rep.

The key to this exercise is maintaining your balance as you lower yourself to the ground on one leg. Feel free to adjust your arms and legs as you see fit to maintain your balance. Try for 50 reps or until fatigued, then switch legs.

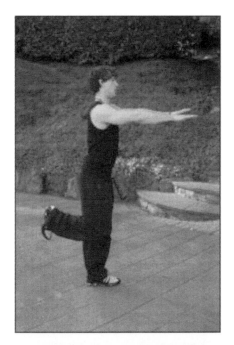

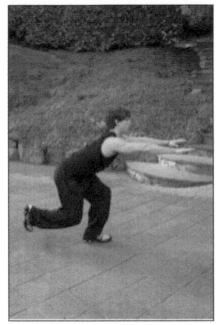

One Leg Front Squats

This exercise is similar to the one leg back squats, except your leg is in front of you. A big difference though is that the extended leg should never touch the ground. Again, this exercise builds real leg strength and balance.

1. Begin standing straight up with your arms crossed in front of your chest.
2. Raise one of your legs off the ground. Try to keep it straight.
3. Slowly begin to bend the standing leg at the knee, lowering your body to the floor. Go as far as you can. Keep in mind the extended leg should NOT touch the ground.
4. Push yourself back up again.

Inhale as you go down, inhale as you come up. Shoot for 50 reps or until fatigued, then switch legs.

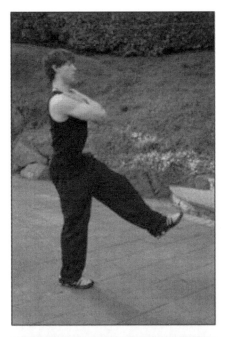

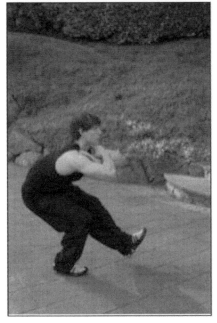

Hindu Jumper Squats

Hindu jumper squats are a more advanced form of regular hindu squats. They can be performed by themselves or with regular hindus. They are really a bodyweight workout in and of themselves and will have you breathing hard in no time.

1. Begin like you're going to perform a standard hindu squat. Stand straight with your arms hanging loosely by your sides.
2. Jump forward 6 inches. Do not jump as high as you can. Simply jump enough to propel your body forward 6 inches.
3. Land with your knees bent.
4. Bend your knees and perform a full squat. If you can you want to keep your hands behind your back as Karen does here. However, if you're taller, you may find that you'll pitch forward. If this is the case, keeping your arms by your side is fine. In either instance, try and keep your back as straight as possible.
5. Jump out of the squat, propelling yourself backwards 6 inches and exhale as you swing your arms upward and then pull them backward.
6. You should now be back in position #1

Repeat this motion until fatigued. If you work at it you will soon be able to perform 100 of these in one go. One good way is to split them up with regular hindu squats. For example, perform 80 hindu squats, followed by 20 jumper squats.

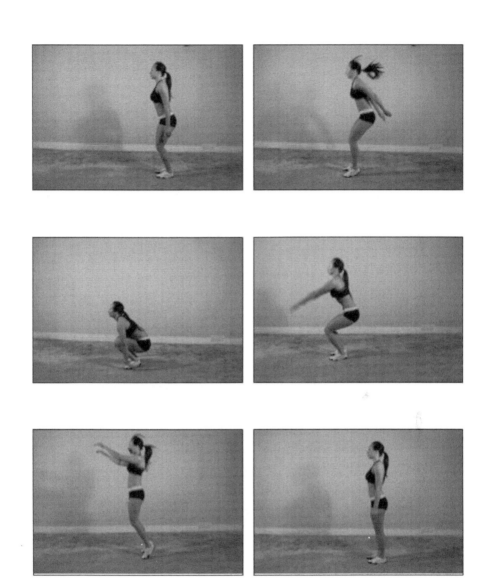

Back Bending Variations

Kneeling Back Arch

This exercise really works your back as well as your abs and butt.

1. Kneel on the floor with your arms and thighs at 90 degree angles to your body.
2. Look up and allow your back to slump downward. Hold this position for 10 seconds.
3. Let your head slump forward and arch your back upwards. Again hold for 10 seconds.
4. Repeat 5 – 10 times.

This stretch should be performed slowly and deliberately. Ensure that your weight is evenly distributed between your knees and hands.

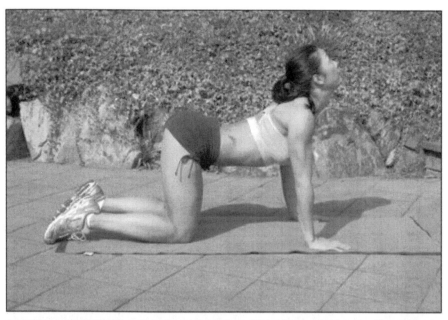

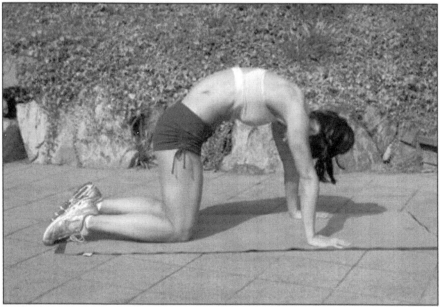

Floor Bow Posture

This exercise is most often seen in yoga classes. It really stretches and strengthens the muscles in your back while increasing the flexibility of your spine.

1. Lie flat on the floor with your stomach on the ground.
2. Bend your legs backward so that you can grab the outside of your feet with your hands. Bend you head backward so that you are looking at the ceiling.
3. Kick upward and backward with your legs. It is this force that will lift your legs and chest off the ground. You are not pulling on your feet with your hands. Think of them as ropes. They are simply there to prevent you from kicking your feet back to the ground.

Hold this position for about five slow, deep breaths.

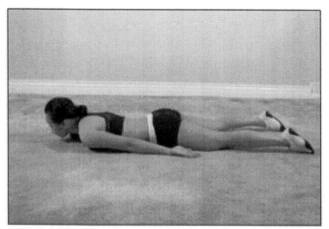

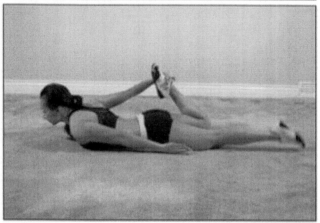

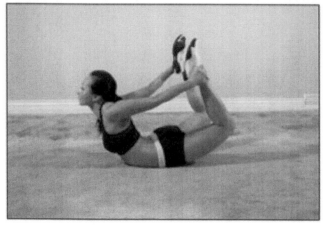

Dynamic Lion Stretch

1. Begin on all fours with your hands slightly wider than shoulder width in front of you and your feet double shoulder width behind you. Both your arms and legs should be straight.
2. Press back with your hands so that you are looking at a spot between your legs while keeping your back straight.
3. Keeping your arms and legs straight come forward so that you arch your back and you are looking at the ceiling.
4. Go back and forth like this 10 times.

Additional Notes

This stretch is essentially a variation of the hindu pushup. The main difference is that you are keeping your arms straight.

This is a great stretch for your shoulders, hips and spine.

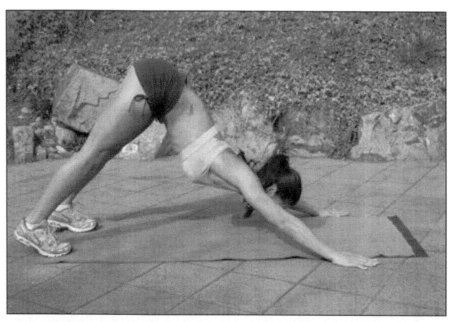

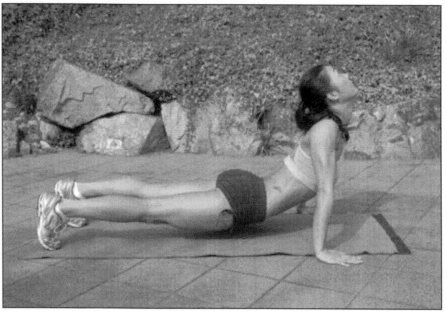

Wall Walking

This is another great exercise that really stretches your spine. When people start learning the back bridge, this is often the exercise that they start with. The backward bending motion really works your abdominals as they will be forced to contract. If you feel a twinge in your back after doing an activity like shoveling snow, a little wall walking is often just the thing to fix you up.

1. Stand with your heels and back flat against a bare wall.
2. Take three or four heel-to-toe steps forward from the wall. (As you get better at this exercise and improve your flexibility, you can take less).
3. Raise your hands upward, palm toward the wall, and start to bend backward.
4. Both hands should touch the wall with your fingertips pointing toward the floor.
5. Slowly walk your hands down the wall. This can feel very awkward at first. Just breathe deeply and calmly and work with gravity as your head approaches the floor.
6. Keep going until your forehead lightly touches the ground.

Once you are in this position you have a choice, you can either: A) turn to your stomach and stand up again, or B) walk back up the wall with your hands.

Make sure you breathe naturally and slowly throughout this exercise. Five to ten repetitions is usually plenty. After completing this exercise, it is often a good idea to stand and bend forward from the waist to stretch your spine in the opposite direction.

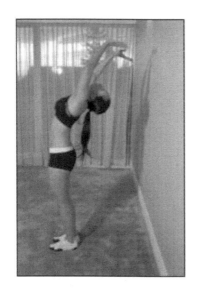 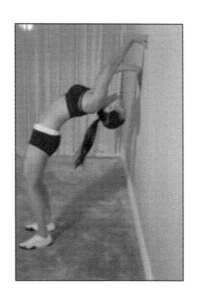

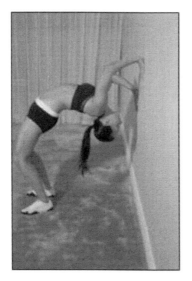 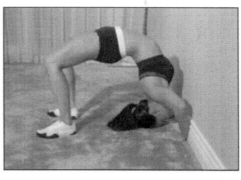

Additional Exercises

Inner Thigh Muscle Raise

This exercise really works the inner thigh muscle, otherwise known as the abductor.

1. Lie on your side, crossing and slightly bending your top leg over your bottom one. Be sure not to let your hips roll back. Make sure you stay aligned on your side.
2. Slowly lift your bottom leg as high as you can, and then lower it gradually.

Try for between 5 and 10 reps, then repeat with the opposite leg.

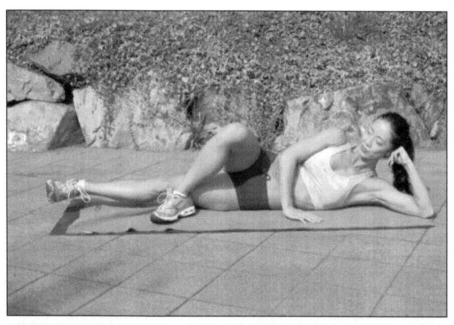

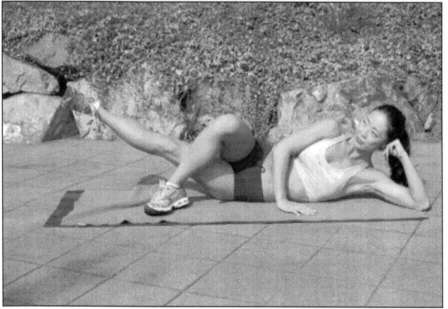

Mountain Climbers

This exercise really works the thighs, buttocks, hips, and abdominals while simultaneously developing tremendous lung power and stamina.

1. Begin on the ground on all fours in a push-up like position.
2. Lift your right foot and bring your right knee under your chest.
3. Without missing a beat return your right foot to the starting position while simultaneously bringing the left knee under your chest. Continue in this fashion without stopping.

Aim to do between 25 and 100 repetitions of this exercise. Remember to breathe naturally at all times.

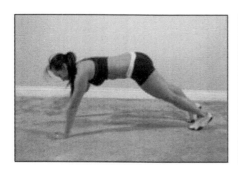 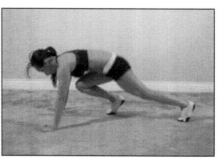

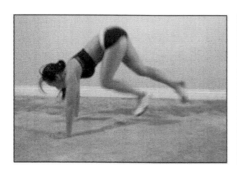 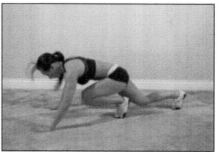

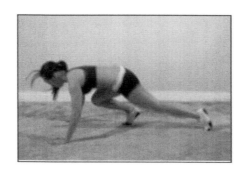

Tai Chi Waist Turner

I generally do this exercise every morning. Not only does it increase the flexibility in your waist and spine but it also massages your internal organs and can help you reduce your waistline.

1. Stand straight with your feet shoulder width apart. Let your arms hang loosely by your sides.
2. Keeping your feet planted start to turn your body to one side, then the other. Let the centrifugal force that you are generating swing your arms as opposed to moving them intentionally in a swinging motion.
3. Each time you have twisted to one side as far as you can comfortably go pause for an instant and let your hands gently slap the kidney area. This will give them a gentle massage.

Remember to breathe naturally as you perform this exercise. Do 50 to 100 repetitions of this exercise everyday.

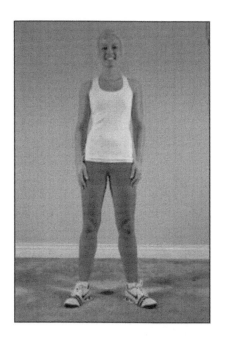

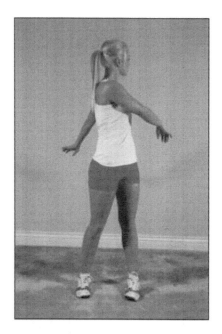

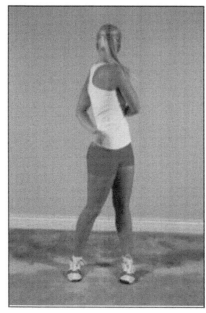

Side Bends

Side bends are a great workout routine for strengthening and stretching the side of your waist.

1. Begin by standing straight with your hands by your sides. If you're tall, you may want to start with your feet shoulder width apart for greater balance later on.
2. Raise your right arm into the air.
3. Start bending your body from the waist to the left. Go as far as you can go.
4. Move back and forth a few inches, bending at the waist from the right to the left. Repeat this slight movement 50 to 100 times. You should really feel this on the side of your waist.
5. Reverse the movement by raising your left arm while you bend at your waist to the right. Again, move back and forth a few inches on your right side 50 to 100 times.

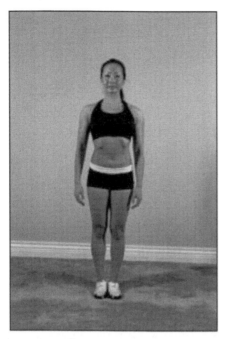 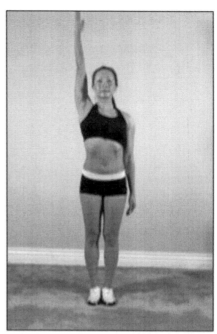

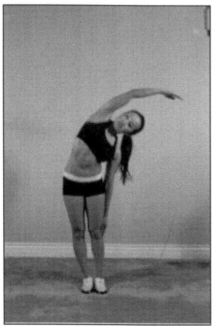 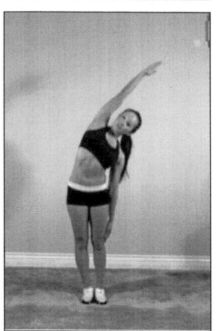

Sideward Leg Lifts

If you want to develop flexibility and strength in the hips and thighs give sideward leg lifts a try.

1. Lie on your side with your legs together.
2. Lift both legs off the floor at the same time. Inhale as you lift them up, exhale as you lower them to the floor.

Do this exercise until fatigued.

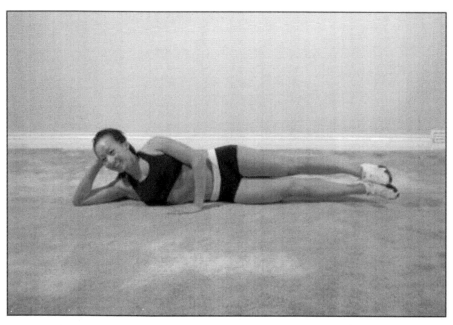

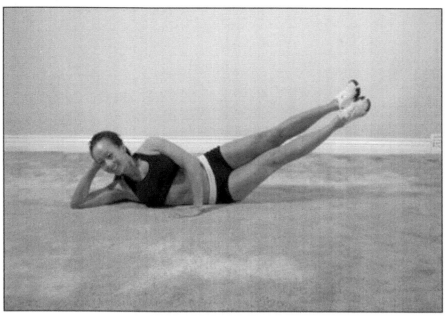

Side Plank Ups

This exercise really works your hip flexors and obliques.

1. Start off by laying on your side on the ground.
2. Prop your right elbow under your shoulder with your legs straight and your hips on the ground.
3. Contract your abdominals as you exhale and raise your hips off the ground. You want to try and make the side of your body as straight as possible. Hold for a second before lowering your hip to the ground.

Aim for 10 repetitions on the right side, then turn over and repeat on the left side.

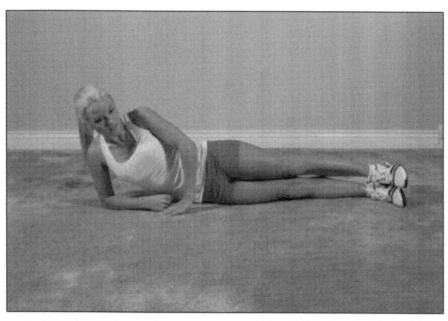

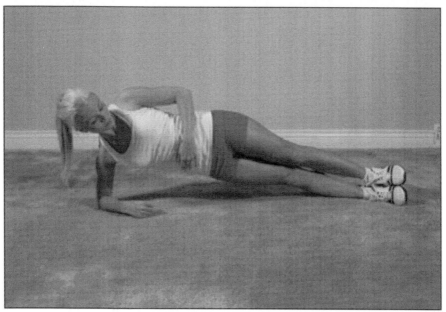

The Table Maker

Performing the table maker will promote flexibility in your spine while building strength in your back, triceps, shoulders, hips and buttocks.

1. Sit down on the floor with your feet straight in front of you and your back perpendicular to the floor.
2. Put the palms of your hands on the floor and push your body forward until the soles of your feet are flat on the ground. Arch your hips and back and let your head fall backward.
3. Squeeze your butt tightly as you straighten your back as much as you can. Your arms and lower legs should now be at 90 degree angles to your body and upper legs.
4. Hold yourself in this table position for a moment, then lower yourself back to the starting position.

Try to perform 10 to 20 repetitions of this exercise. Inhale as you push yourself up, exhale down.

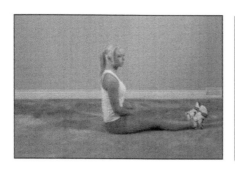

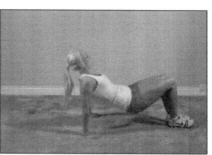

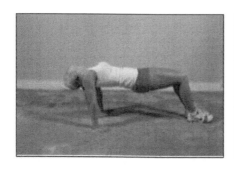

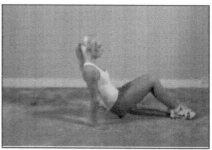

The Stretcher

This exercise is a more difficult variation of the table maker. When you've mastered the table maker, try the stretcher on for size.

1. Just like the table maker begin on the floor with your legs out straight and your hands palm down at your sides.
2. Push your body forward so that your feet are flat on the ground while keeping your legs straight. Arch your hips and back. Keep both your legs and back as straight as possible.
3. Hold this position for a beat, then lower yourself gently to the floor.

You should aim to do 10 to 20 repetitions of this exercise. Inhale as you raise yourself up, exhale on the way down.

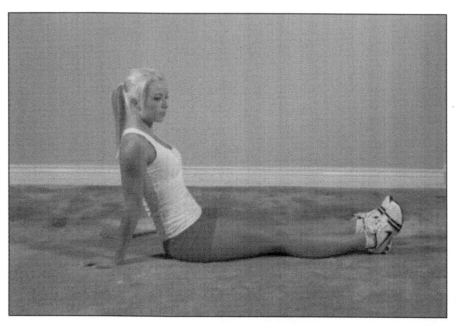

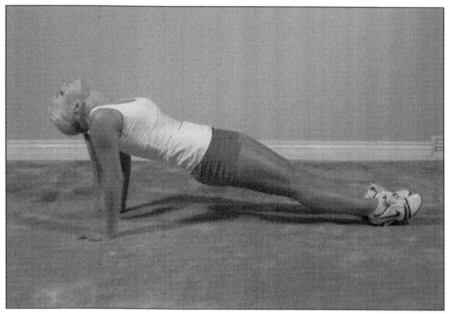

No Momentum Sit-Ups

What makes these sit-ups so effective is that it's almost impossible to cheat when doing them. You can't use momentum or pull on your head or neck to get yourself up. This exercise really strengthens your abdominals, lower back, and hip flexors. Another name for this exercise is vampire risers as you can pretend that you're one of the living dead rising slowly from their grave while performing it.

1. Lie down flat on the floor with straight legs. Your arms should be by your side with your palms flat on the floor.
2. Slowly start to raise your upper body using your abdominal muscles only. Your heels and legs should never come off the floor.
3. Come up all the way until your upper body is perpendicular to the floor.
4. Reverse direction and slowly return to the starting position. Go slowly here as well as you want to work your muscles going in both directions.

Do as many as you can. Remember to inhale on your way up and exhale on your way down. If you wish to make the exercise harder, you can keep your arms by your sides instead of lifting them out in front of you.

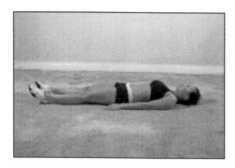 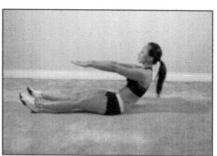

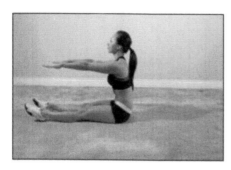 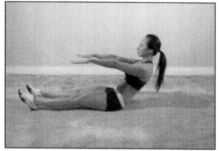

Butt Lift Leg Raise

This is an interesting exercise that will really work your lower body.

1. Lie flat on your back with your right knee bent while your left leg remains straight.
2. With your arms by your sides lift and extend your left leg. However, you want to keep both knees together at the same time.
3. Lift your butt of the floor about 3 to 6 inches while keeping your thighs parallel to each other.
4. Hold briefly, then lower your body to the floor, keeping your left leg extended the whole time.

Perform this motion 10 times on the one side. Then rest and repeat the motion with your right leg.

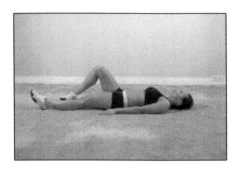 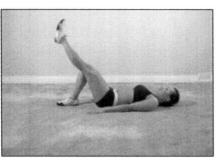

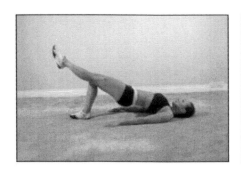 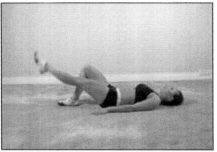

Leg Lifts Behind Head

This exercise will not only strengthen your abdominals, lower back and hip flexors, but it will also give your spine, shoulders and upper back a nice stretch. Like all abdominal exercises it will also massage your internal organs while increasing your circulation and aiding the digestive process.

1. Lie down flat with your back on the floor and your arms by your sides.
2. Lift your head so that your chin is almost touching your chest.
3. While keeping your head up start lifting your legs as straight as possible into the air.
4. Continue to raise your legs until your toes touch the floor behind your head.
5. Lower your legs back to the ground, letting them softly touch the floor.

Inhale as you raise your legs, exhale as you lower them. Do as many repetitions as you can.

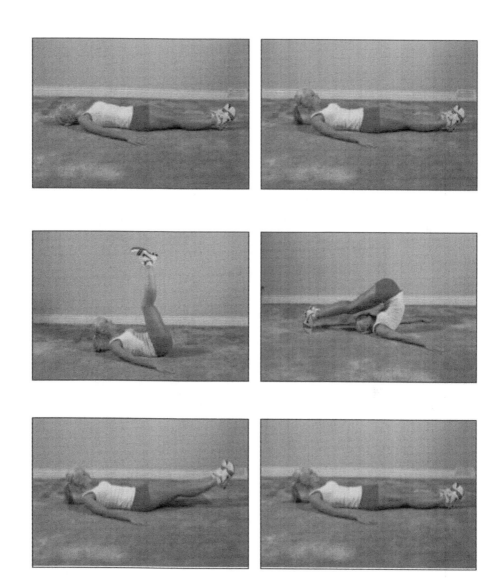

Plank Butt Ups

This exercise really hits your core, including your abdominals and butt.

1. Start off by laying face down on the ground.
2. Prop your elbows under your shoulders and rise up on your toes. Only your forearms and toes should be touching the ground.
3. Squeeze your abdominals tightly as you lift your butt up toward the ceiling while rising up on your toes. Hold for a second then lower yourself to the starting position.

At no time during this exercise should your back sag downward toward the floor. Try and do 10 repetitions of this exercise.

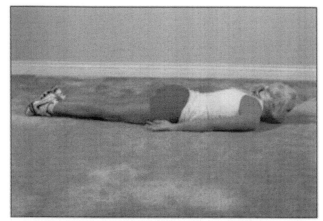

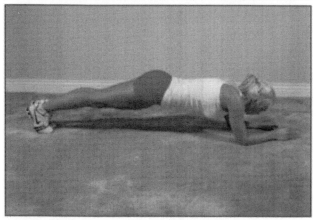

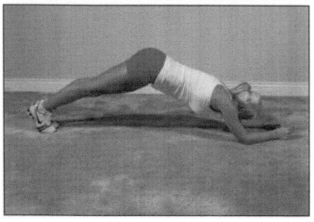

Front Bridge

Once you're able to hold a hands-free back bridge for 3 minutes straight, it's a good idea to perform a front bridge to balance things out a bit.

1. Squat down on all fours. If you are on a hard surface you will want to place a mat or soft towel above your head. In this picture we did not, as the surface was soft. However, if you sweat a lot you may still want to use a towel.
2. Place your forehead on the ground in front of you.
3. Extend your legs so that they are straight and your feet form a triangle with the top of you head.
4. Tuck your chin in until it touches the top of your chest and then place your hands behind your back.

Breathe slowly and deeply through your nose. Eventually, your goal is to hold this position for three minutes.

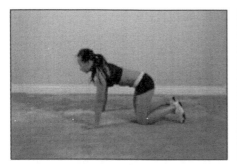 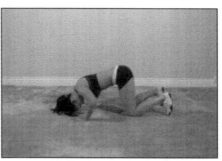

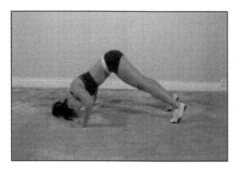 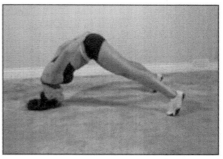

The Rower

This is a great exercise for building strength in your abdominals and core.

1. Lay flat on the ground with your legs straight and your arms by your sides.
2. Tuck your chin into your chest. Tighten your stomach and press your lower back into the ground.
3. Sit up and swing your arms forward while at the same time bringing your knees into your chest.
4. Bring your knees in as close to your chest as possible while keeping your arms straight.

Reverse the movement until you return to the starting position. Always perform this exercise at a controlled and moderate pace.

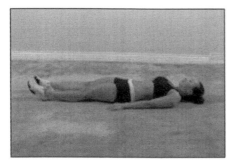 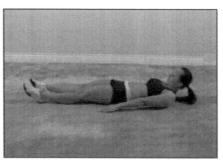

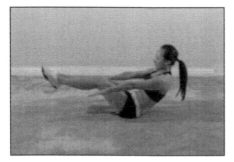 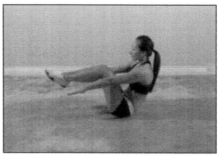

Leg Scissors

This exercise really hits your inner and outer thighs, hip flexors, and abdominals.

1. Lie down flat on your back with your legs straight and your arms by your side.
2. Tuck your chin in to your chest while you lift both legs about 6 inches off the floor. Your legs can either be straight or slightly bent.
3. Inhale as you open your legs wide.
4. Exhale as you reverse direction and cross your legs.

For this exercise, shoot for between 25 and 50 repetitions. Remember to alternate the leg that goes under and over on each repetition.

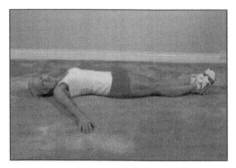 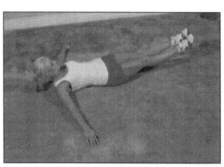

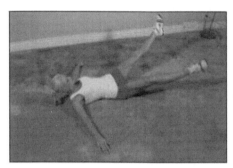 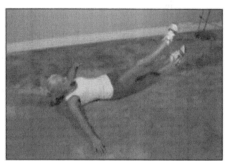

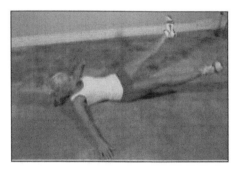 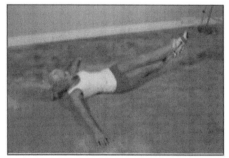

119

6 Inch Crunch

This is another great exercise for your abdominals and hip flexors.

1. Lie down on the floor with your arms crossed on your chest. You should be flat on your back with your legs straight.
2. Concentrate on pushing the small of your back toward the floor while you raise your legs 6 inches off the ground.
3. Tuck your chin into your chest. Now, keep your legs raised while you exhale and contract your abdominal muscles. Try to pull your bottom rib toward your hip.
4. Relax and lower your upper body back to the floor without dropping your legs. Try doing this 20 times while keeping your legs in the air.

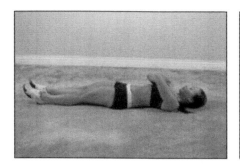 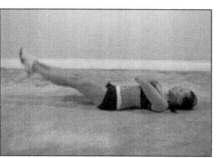

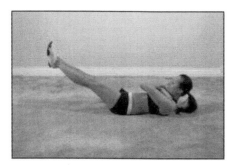 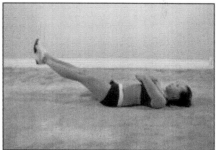

Ab Infinities

This exercise really works your abdominals, oblique muscles and hip flexors.

1. Lie flat on your back with your arms by your sides and your legs straight.
2. Raise your chin to your chest as you simultaneously raise your legs about six inches above the floor. Use your arms for balance.

3. Use your legs to draw the infinity symbol "∞" in the air.

When doing this exercise go first in one direction. Once you've completed one infinity symbol, reverse direction and go the opposite way.

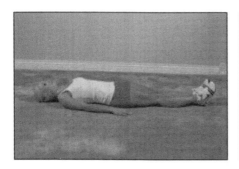 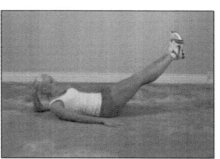

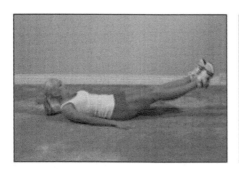 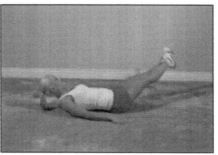

Reverse Leg Lifts

This bodyweight exercise gives your lower back a good stretch while also strengthening your abdominals, lower back, and buttocks.

1. Lie flat on the floor, face down, with your arms stretched forward.
2. Take a deep inhale and lift both legs at the same time. Hold of a couple of seconds.
3. Exhale your breath and lower your legs to the floor.

Keep you nose to the floor as you lift your legs in order to protect your back. You can bend your knees slightly if you wish.

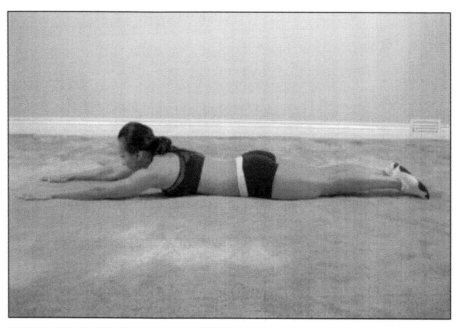

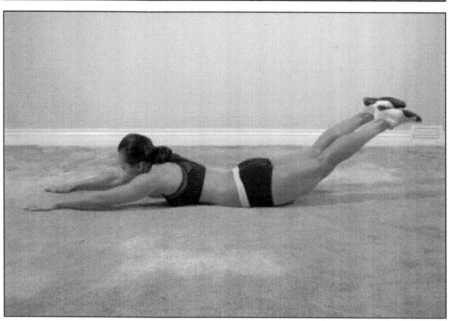

Torso Lifts

Torso lifts are the opposite of the leg lifts. You'll be surprised how much your abdominals, hips, and back are worked in this exercise. Plus, you get to pretend that you're Superman or Superwoman, which is kind of fun ;)

1. Lie face down on the floor with your arms stretched forward.
2. Keeping your legs on the ground, inhale and lift your arms, chest, and abdominals as high as you can. Hold for a second.
3. Exhale and lower yourself to the floor.

Try to perform this exercise 10 times at a minimum.

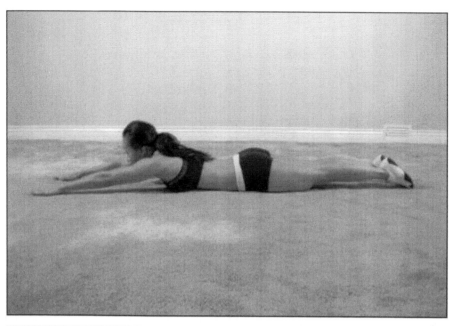

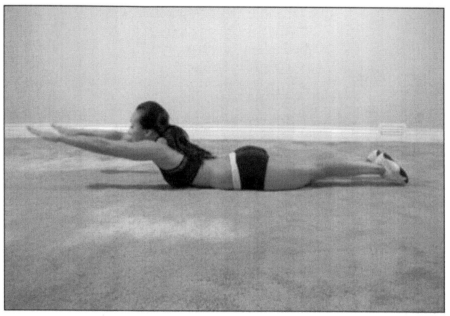

Headstand Hold

Performing a headstand can be challenging at first but the benefits you gain are substantial. Not only does it improve your balance and confidence it also allows extra blood to reach your brain. This will help you feel refreshed and powerful.

1. Place a cushion or mat in front of you where you will rest your head if the surface you are on is hard (the carpet here is soft, so it wasn't needed here). If you don't have a mat a large folded towel will work well also. You just want to be comfortable. Start standing about a foot from the wall.
2. Squat down and place your head on the mat and your hands on the floor. Your head and hands should perform a triangle.
3. Bring your right knee under your chest.
4. Kick up with your left leg while you push off the floor with your right foot.
5. Straighten your legs.

Breathe deeply and calmly through your nose throughout this posture. Try and hold this position for 30 seconds at first. From there try working up to a full minute and beyond.

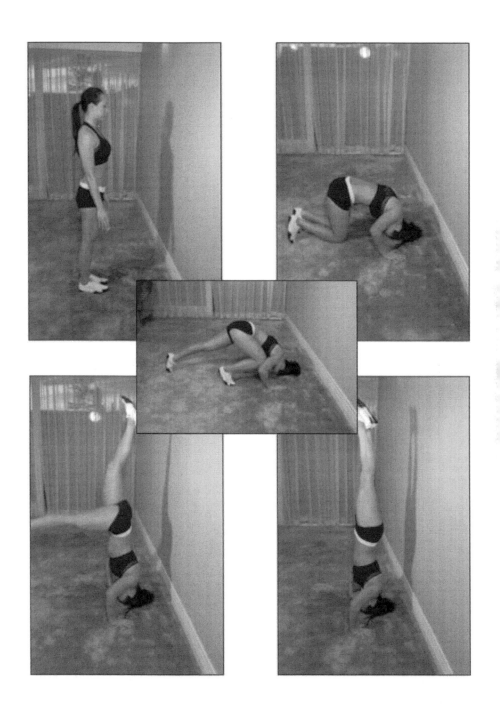

V-Ups

V-ups are a great ab exercise as they hit both the upper and lower abdominals at the same time.

1. Lie flat on your back with your legs straight and your arms by your sides.
2. Exhale while you raise your legs up about 45 degrees while reaching toward your toes with your arms.
3. Try and touch your hands to your feet. You should be balancing on your butt at this point.
4. Slowly lower yourself to the starting position.

Always perform this exercise in a controlled motion without swinging your legs or jerking your upper body. Aim to do 10 repetitions at a minimum.

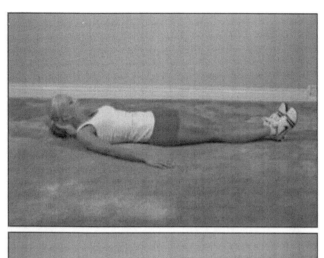

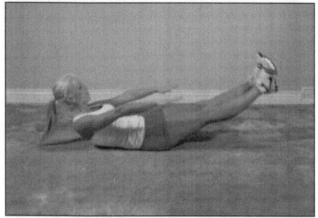

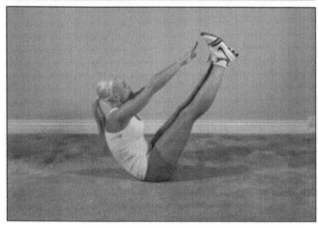

Headstand Leg Tuck

Headstands are a terrific example of bodyweight training as they force you to maintain your balance which works your entire body. Your brain will also be invigorated by the extra blood it will receive while being in the inverted position.

1. Place a folded towel or pillow in front of a wall for cushioning if you are on a hard surface.
2. Squat down and place your forehead in the palm of your hands. Let your elbows come out so that they form a triangle on the floor with your head.
3. Place your knees on your elbows and slowly lift your feet off the ground. Your legs should form a 90 degree angle.
4. Exhale your breath as you raise your legs into an extended position. Do this slowly and in a controlled fashion. Imagine yourself "blowing up" your legs.
5. Hold for a second at the top, then lower your legs to the 90 degree angle in step 3.
6. Repeat 10 times or more if desired.

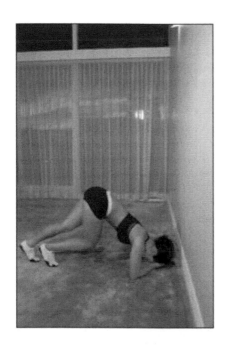

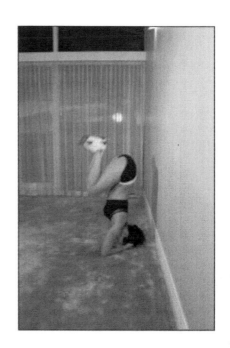

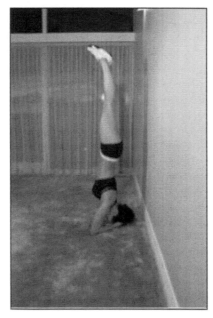

Push Up and Inverted Crunch

This exercise gives you all of the benefits of a regular pushup while really hitting your abs at the same time.

1. Assume the standard pushup position.
2. Keeping your back straight, lower your body to the floor.
3. Push yourself back up again.
4. Again keeping your back straight, bring your left knee forward.
5. Bring your left knee back.
6. Bring your right leg forward until it touches your right elbow.
7. Bring your right knee back, then go back to step #2. Continue until fatigued.

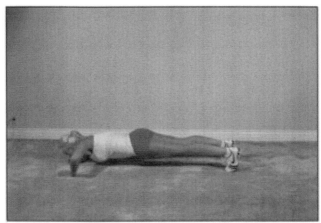

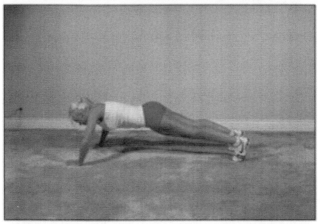

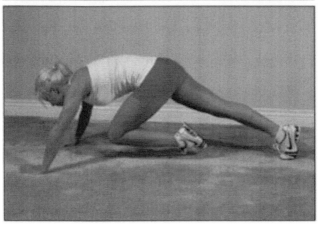

Reverse Handstand

The reverse handstand builds tremendous strength in your shoulders, back, and arms. I prefer it to a regular handstand as you are able to use the wall to "walk" up into position as opposed to kicking up. Try and hold this position for a minute at first. From there shoot for 3 minutes. The sky's really the limit with these kinds of exercises. You can always do more (if you want to).

1. Assume a pushup position with your feet touching the wall. Place one of your feet on the wall.
2. Start walking backwards on your hands, while simultaneously walking up the wall with your feet. Keep going until your chest is flat against the wall.
3. From this position simply breathe deeply and hold it for as long as you can.

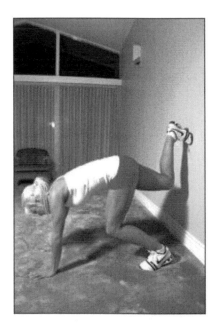

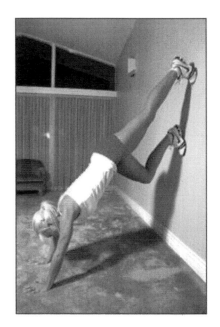

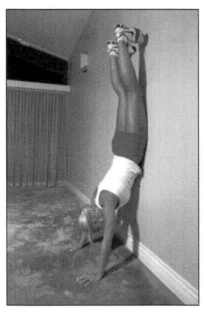

Handstand Walkout

This is an interesting variation of the regular reverse handstand. The walking out portion really works your arms and shoulders.

1. Assume a pushup position with your feet touching the wall.
2. Start walking backwards on your hands while simultaneously walking up the wall with your feet.
3. Keep walking backwards until you are performing a handstand flush against the wall.
4. From this reverse handstand position, walk your hands forward until your body forms a 45 degree angle with the floor.   Your body should be straight and rigid.
5. Once here, walk your body backward again until you are in the reverse handstand position. Continue in this fashion until fatigued.

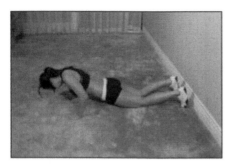 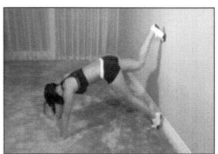

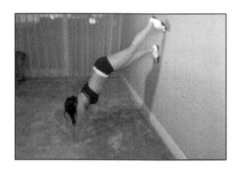 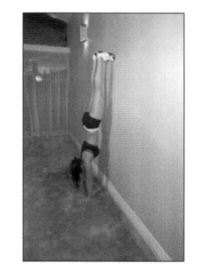

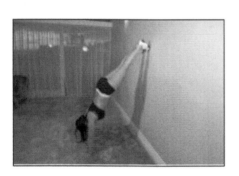

139

Clock Walking

This is a fun but tough bodyweight exercise that really works your upper body. In it you pretend you're a minute hand on a clock. Here's what you do.

1. Get into a basic pushup position and hold. Make sure that your feet are close together and your arms are locked out.
2. Start walking your hands in a circle while keeping your feet stationary. If your head is at the 12 o'clock position, keep walking until your hands are at the 6 o'clock position. Then walk your hands back the other way until you're back to 12 o'clock. This counts as one repetition.

Try for between three and ten repetitions. If this is too easy for you, try performing a full 360° around before coming back.

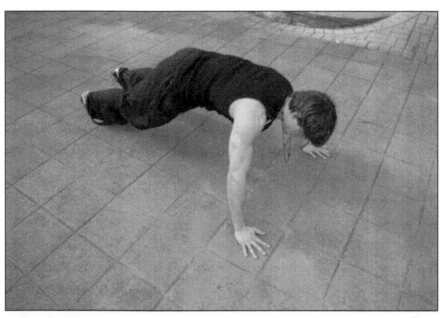

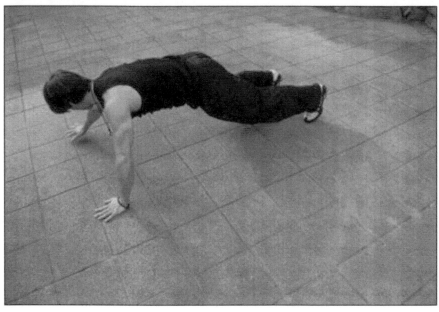

Workout Routines

What follows are some additional workout routines that you may wish to try. Enjoy!

Advanced Natural Fitness Workout

If you're getting really good and desire a level of fitness and health that few possess, try working up to the below:

500 Hindu Squats

100 Hindu Pushups

10 Finger Tip Pushups

10 Reverse Pushups

20 Ab Infinities

20 reps of the Rower

3 Minute Back Bridge

With this advanced workout, the thing you'll notice most is the 500 Hindu Squats. I know this seems like a lot but it can be done (I actually did 1000 a couple of times). There is no difference between working your way up to 50 as there is to 500. Just get started, working on them everyday and increasing your work load by one. You should be able to do 500 in less than 15 minutes if you are going at a good clip.

Once again,there is no need for you to get to this level unless you want to (or maybe if you're a firefighter / police officer and lives are on the line). I'm offering this as a suggestion only. If you only do the basic workout and nothing else you'll be fitter than 95% of the people out there.

Deck Of Cards Workout

I usually try to avoid workout routines that require any kind equipment at all. However, for this workout all you need is a deck of cards. Here's what you do. Pick any four exercises from this book and assign them a card suit. For example:

1. Hindu Squats - Diamonds
2. Hindu Pushups - Hearts
3. Leg Scissors - Spades
4. V - Ups - Clubs

Now all you do is shuffle the deck and start dealing the cards one at a time. If you deal a 5 of diamonds perform 5 Hindu squats. If you get a 7 of spades perform 7 leg scissors. For the face cards assign them a value of between 10 and 15, depending on your fitness level. For the times I've done this, I've used the jokers as well for back bridging. Try it. It's a great workout.

200 Pushup Workout

If you like pushups and want to build tremendous upper body strength, this is the workout for you.

3 minutes Back Bridge

100 Hindu Squats

50 Hindu Pushups

10 Elevated Pike Pushups

10 Pike Pushups

20 Finger Tip Pushups

10 Reverse Pushups

25 Hindu Pushups (with feet wide apart)

25 Hindu Pushups (with feet close together)

25 Atlas Pushups

Wall Workout

You'll need a bare wall to perform this workout. It will really build up your upper body but you might scuff up your wall a bit in the process. The hindu squats at the end are for your cardio.

1 minute reverse handstand 3 times. Rest no more than 1 minute between sets

10 handstand walkouts

5 walkout pushups

Wall walking and hold as long as you can in a back bridge (work up to 3 minutes)

100 Hindu Squats

Ladder Workouts

Ladder workouts were originally used by Soviet athletes before the iron curtain fell. The idea is to perform the same exercise for many sets but never to the point of failure. An example of this would be an athlete who performs 30 pushups every hour while he (or she) is awake. If this person get up at 7 and goes to bed at 10:00, they would be awake for 15 hours. This means they would be performing 450 pushups for that day. In theory you could do this workout for weeks and weeks, never get tired, yet still gain incredible strength. The workout below does not stretch on throughout the day, but the principle is the same.

3 minute Back Bridge

20 Hindu Pushups + 20 Hindu Squats

rest for 40 seconds

20 Atlas Pushups + 20 Hindu Squats

rest for 40 seconds

20 Hindu Pushups + 20 Hindu Squats

rest for 40 seconds

20 Reverse Pushups + 20 Hindu Squats

rest for 40 seconds

20 Hindu Pushups + 20 Hindu Squats

rest for 40 seconds

20 Fingertip Pushups + 20 Hindu Squats

rest for 40 seconds

20 Hindu Pushups + 20 Hindu Squats

rest for 40 seconds

20 Pike Pushups + 20 Hindu Squats

rest for 40 seconds

20 Hindu Pushups + 20 Hindu Squats

rest for 40 seconds

20 Reverse Pushups + 20 Hindu Squats

When you finish this workout, you'll have done 200 pushups and 200 Hindu Squats in less than 25 minutes. If you wish to make it tougher you can reduce the rest period between the sets.

Jumping Rope With Pushups

If you only have 15 minutes, here's a great workout you can do. All you need is a jump rope (and the ability to use it, of course).

Begin by jumping rope for 200 repetitions.

Do 25 Hindu pushups

Jump rope for another 200 repetitions

Do 25 regular pushups with your elbows close to our body

Jump rope for another 200 reps

Do 25 Hindu pushups

Jump rope for another 200 reps

Do 25 regular pushups with your hands wide

Jump rope for a final 200 reps

To make it even harder, you can always add to the number of pushups you're doing.

Cardiovascular Exercises

When it comes to cardiovascular fitness performing exercises like Hindu squats and pushups are really all you need, so long as they're performed at a brisk pace. However, if you wish to do more, I would recommend two exercises: jumping rope and hill sprints. Both are high intensity exercises that take relatively little time to complete. In my mind this is why they are "animal-like" and are so healthy for you.

In the wild, animals either walk at a relaxed pace or run as fast as they can over short distances (typically to get food or to avoid being eaten). They don't run over long distances at a medium pace for no reason at all. By exercising in this way animals are able to build incredible endurance and lung power. If it works for them, it'll work for us too.

Need some evidence? Think of Olympic athletes. The bodies of the sprinters are lean and powerful. They are as healthy as human beings can be. On the other hand the athletes who participate in the long distance events, although healthy, do not look nearly as good. Although it's true they have no fat on them, they have far less muscle than the sprinters. Long distance running wears your body down. It breaks down muscle tissue, harms your joints, and prematurely ages you. If you want to be as healthy as an animal you want to focus on high intensity movements for short periods. This is why I recommend jumping rope and hill sprints. Try them out. I think you'll be surprised at just how effective they are.

Jumping Rope

Jumping rope has long been considered one of the best cardiovascular exercises in existence. Many athletes, but especially boxers, have always made skipping rope a cornerstone of their bodyweight training routines. Why? Because it works! Not only does skipping rope give your lungs a great workout but it also works your legs, abdomen, chest, shoulders, back and arms. It's been said that 10 minutes of skipping rope is the equivalent of 30 minutes of hard running. From my experience, I believe this is accurate. If you really want to get in great cardiovascular shape try the routine below:

1. One minute - Jump Rope as FAST as you are able
2. 30 seconds rest
3. Two minutes - Jump Rope as FAST as you can.
4. One minute rest
5. Three minutes - Jump Rope as FAST as you can.
6. One minute rest
7. Two minutes - Jump Rope as FAST as you can.
8. 30 seconds rest
9. One minute - Jump Rope as FAST as you are able

I know this routine looks simple, but I assure you, it isn't. If you've never jumped rope before simply do what you can. If you can only skip for one minute, then do that. It's a great start. If you practice your rope skipping at least three times a week you'll be surprised how fast your endurance builds up and how soon you'll be able to do the full routine.

Hill Sprints

Hill sprints are an amazing exercise for building lung power, strength, and endurance. NFL running backs frequently use hill sprints to help them build their explosive speed, power, and endurance. Unlike long distance running, hill sprints actually help you build muscle, as opposed to wearing your muscle away.

Again, this exercise is really only for those who want to be hyper fit. It is not an easy exercise. I remember the first time I tried it I nearly threw up in some poor persons rose garden after only two sprints. As with all of these exercises, do what you can do at first. Keep at it, and try and do a little more each time.

To perform this exercise find a hill with a gently increasing gradient. If you live in a flat area you can perform this exercise on stairs. The stairs in a football stadium would work nicely. At any rate, start at the bottom of the hill and then sprint as fast as you can for between 10 and no more than 30 seconds. Once you've finished your sprint, walk back down the hill to your starting point, catching your breath as you do so. As soon as you reach the bottom, sprint back up the hill and repeat the process.

From my experience performing 5 hills sprints in this fashion is plenty, although you can do more if you choose. However, hill sprints are very intense. I do not recommend performing them everyday. You are better off performing them every other day in order to give your body some rest.

About the Author

David Nordmark has a life long interest in health and fitness. In the past he has participated in such sports as soccer, basketball and hockey. He also was once an avid runner and weightlifter, but has since come to his senses. Today he mainly does natural exercises like Yoga and the Body Weight exercises found on his website, www.animal-kingdom-workouts.com.

He currently lives in beautiful Vancouver, British Columbia Canada, although he really wouldn't mind living somewhere else during the winter. He's currently working on making that dream a reality.

If you have any questions for him, feel free to contact him using the contact form which can be found on this website. Here's the link:

http://www.animal-kingdom-workouts.com/contactme.html

About the Models

Kerry Diotte is a Vancouver-based model who enjoys exercise and playing soccer. She is available for fitness, glamour, and commercial modeling work. She can be reached at kerrydiotte05@msn.com. To view her portfolio, visit

http://www.modelmayhem.com/633989.

Karen Pang is a Vancouver-based fitness model and competitor. She also travels frequently to Los Angeles and Toronto. She is available for fitness modeling, glamour and bikini shoots. She can be reached at karen@misskarenpang.com or through her website at www.misskarenpang.com. To view her portfolio, visit

 http://www.modelmayhem.com/558190

Christine Chou is a Vancouver-based fitness competitor. She can be reached at chrischou_@hotmail.com or through her website at

http://fitfabfoodies.com/

Dylan Hickey is a Vancouver-based personal trainer and model. He can be reached at dylan_hickey11@hotmail.com or through his website at

http://www.freeworkoutguides.com/

One Last Thing

I just wanted to thank you again for purchasing my book. I sincerely hope that you found it interesting and worthwhile.

Finally, if you did enjoy it I'd like to ask you for a favor. If you would you be kind enough to leave a review for this book on amazon or wherever you purchased it from it would be greatly appreciated.

Thank you in advance and I wish you all the best in the future!

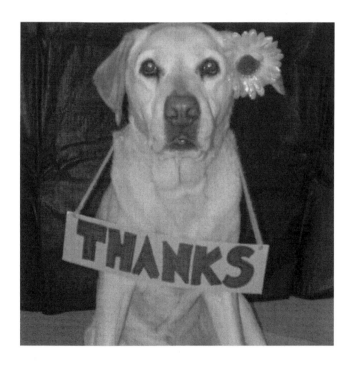

Also By David Nordmark

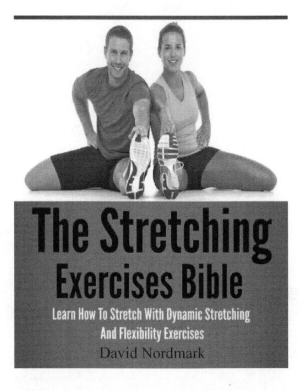

The Stretching Exercises Bible

Do you want to learn how to increase your Strength, Flexibility, Stamina and Energy Levels Naturally? If so then the Stretching Exercises Bible can help you. Aside from the standard stretching exercises it also contains many unique deep breathing, joint loosening and energy exercises that are designed to get your muscles loose and energy flowing.Buy this book and start feeling better today!

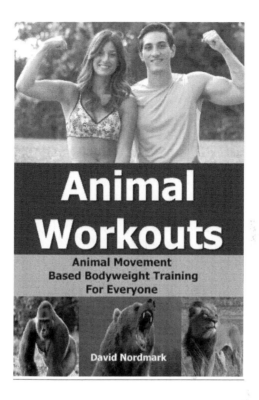

Animal Workouts

Animal Workouts is a fitness program based on natural animal movements. Amazingly effective and fun, these exercises are appropriate for any age and fitness level, require no special equipment and can be done anywhere at anytime. Whether you want to lose belly fat, gain almost superhuman strength or beat the aging process Animal Workouts can help you get there in only minutes a day.

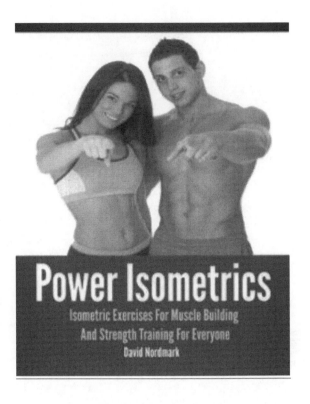

Power Isometrics

Do you want to Burn Fat and Build Muscle from the comfort of your own home quickly and easily using no special equipment whatsoever? If so, Power Isometrics is for you. These time proven exercises can be done anywhere at anytime, are incredibly safe and effective and can give you a full body workout in less than 1/2 an hour a day. Start transforming your body today with Power Isometrics.

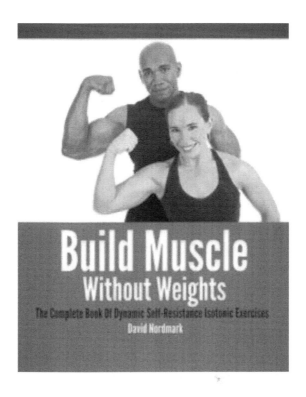

Build Muscle Without Weights

Build Muscle Without Weights is a revolutionary exercise system which utilizes self-resistance isotonic exercises to build muscle and sculpt the body safely and easily. For thousands of years athletes of all kinds have utilized these kinds of exercises, pitting muscle against muscle, to build strong and functional physiques. Order this book and get the body of your dreams today!

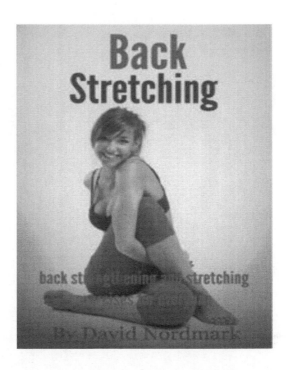

Build Muscle Without Weights

If you suffer from back pain or discomfort you're not alone. We are all likely to suffer from some kind of back pain at least once in our lives. If you've ever felt a twinge in your back after sitting in the office all day or if you've been dealing with back issues of one kind or another all your life Back Stretching is for you. Get ready to say goodbye to back pain, starting today.

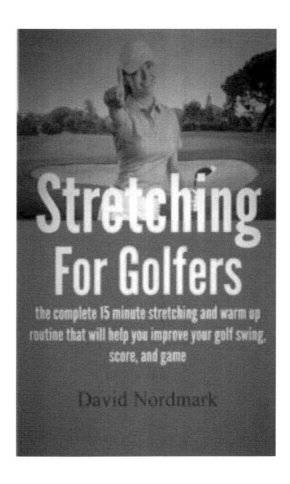

Stretching For Golfers

Being relaxed and flexible is a prerequisite for playing a great game of golf that most recreational golfers ignore. Don't be one of them. Stiff and sore muscles not only detract from your enjoyment of the game but they lower your score as well. Stretching For Golfers provides you with a simple routine that anyone can do that will help improve your game today.

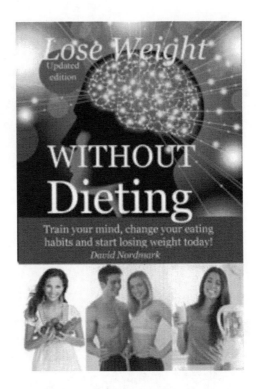

Lose Weight Without Dieting

The key to long-term weight loss is to make permanent changes to your everyday eating habits. This book will help you build a fat loss blueprint that will eradicate your old eating habits and replace them with new positive ones. Overtime you will lose all the weight you want for real, and you'll do it without dieting. Get this book and start changing your body today!

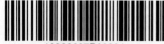

12388697R00091

Printed in Great Britain
by Amazon.co.uk, Ltd.,
Marston Gate.